DISCARD

Substance Use
and Abuse

Substance Use and Abuse

Sociological Perspectives

Victor N. Shaw

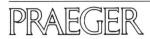

Westport, Connecticut
London

Library of Congress Cataloging-in-Publication Data

Shaw, Victor N.
    Substance use and abuse : sociological perspectives / Victor N. Shaw.
        p.   cm.
    Includes bibliographical references and index.
    ISBN 0–275–97139–2 (alk. paper)
    1. Substance abuse—Social aspects—United States.   I. Title.
HV4999.2.S52   2002
362.29′1′0973—dc21   2002067938

British Library Cataloguing in Publication Data is available.

Library of Congress Catalog Card Number: 2002067938
ISBN: 0–275–97139–2

First published in 2002

Praeger Publishers, 88 Post Road West, Westport, CT 06881
An imprint of Greenwood Publishing Group, Inc.
www.praeger.com

Printed in the United States of America

∞™

The paper used in this book complies with the
Permanent Paper Standard issued by the National
Information Standards Organization (Z39.48–1984).

10 9 8 7 6 5 4

Contents

Introduction

The idea of writing this book developed during my two-year postdoctoral scholarship in substance abuse research at the University of California–Los Angeles, under the auspices of the National Institute on Drug Abuse. As I participated in research projects to witness how data are gathered and analyzed, I soon realized that the field of substance use and abuse is plagued with an outgrowth of unrelated data collection and contingent explanations conceived in response to specific data. As I attended meetings and ploughed through the literature to learn how research findings are interpreted and reported, I gradually became convinced that there is a phenomenal poverty of, and therefore a dire need for, understanding of the fundamental issues in the field.

I then went back to my training in sociology and criminology. I examined the major concepts and theories I learned and found most of them relevant and insightful to my quest for understanding on the matter of substance, substance use, and substance users. I began with the social control perspective, into which I delved deeply while working on my previous book, *Social Control in China*. I tackled about two perspectives a year. After nearly six years of serious intellectual effort, I now have a whole variety of sociological explanations for substance use and abuse, including anomie, career, conflict, functionalist, rational choice, social control, social disorganization, social learning, social reaction, and subculture perspectives.

In form, all perspectives follow a similar logical sequence and have a comparable systematic framework. Sources of inspiration review relevant conceptual and empirical contributions in the existing literature. The theoretical framework builds upon definition, theoretical image, theoretical component, theoretical application, and empirical test. Specifically, definition explains key concepts and presents a miniature view of the perspective. Theoretical image provides a general picture of substance use and abuse, across society and through history, in the spirit of the perspective. Theoretical component addresses major issues inherent in the perspective, such as stages of use, change through stages, and roles of use under the career perspective. Theoretical application proposes challenging topics and opportunities, derivable from the perspective, for further exploration. Empirical test elaborates how conventional research methods can be adapted to carry out concrete research projects using the perspective. There is also a major section dealing with the perspective's policy implications for public health, social control, life and community, and work and organization.

In content, each perspective stands on its own as an independent, self-sufficient theoretical system. First, the anomie perspective looks at substance and substance use as resource, opportunity, or means in people's reaction to their social structural conditions, specifically moral ambiguity or confusion and social strain or depression. As a resource, substance may be used to achieve material success. Substance use may be initiated and sustained to gain social status. As opportunity, substance may be used to excuse failure in life struggle. Substance use may be attempted to escape from active social functioning. As means, substance may be touted as a coping mechanism. Substance use may also be instituted as a routine defense against disappointment, frustration, and stress in personal experience with society. According to the anomie perspective, to reduce substance use and abuse is to improve social conditions so that laws are made clear, accessible, and understandable to common citizens, laws and social norms are enforced fairly and equitably across the population, and, most important, social resources and opportunities are provided equally for all members of the society.

Next, the career perspective compares substance use and abuse to the employment career that features upward and downward mobility over the individual's life span. From a career point of view, substance use is not just use of substance. It is distributed across various stages, from initiation, experimentation, habituation, dependence, problematic experience, assistance seeking, treatment, cessation, relapse, and maturation, to abstinence, in specific career pathways. Substance users are not just users of a common identity. They are differentiated into various roles or statuses through individual careers. In their peculiar use career path, users may experience various changes in physiological, psychological, personal, and social dimensions and take on different perspectives in work and life. Social reactions are usually fashioned accordingly through stages of individual change. For instance, prevention comes typically in the initial phases whereas treatment takes place when individuals develop serious symptoms of addiction.

The conflict perspective detailed in chapter 3 views substance, substance use, and substance users as sites, vehicles, or carriers of division, tension, conflict, or confrontation between or among individuals, groups, institutions, social classes, or other identifiable entities. On the one hand, conflict within and between individuals and groups, social division between the rich and the poor, the powerful and the powerless, or the educated and the uneducated, as well as tension between human beings and non-human existence, may singly or jointly create and maintain conditions for substance use and abuse. On the other hand, substance use divides people into contrasting or opposing groups between addiction and abstinence, between dependency and self-sufficiency, between drug users and drug czars, between those who are in need of help and those who offer professional assistance, as well as between the oppressed, the deprived, the treated, and their oppressing, possessing, intervening counterparts. For example, substance users may challenge long- or widely held beliefs and norms, making themselves natural targets for traditional, conservative, or mainstream criticism and condemnation. They may pose as a possible threat, disruption, or danger to social order, turning themselves into easy prey for criminal justice officials, medical professionals, and service personnel in their respective efforts of punishment, treatment, and rehabilitation.

Chapter 4 focuses on the functionalist perspective and investigates substance use and abuse in the context of the larger system, how substance use and abuse are necessitated by a system, and what they offer to the functional operation, maintenance, and progression of the system. At the abstract level, the functionalist perspective explores how substance may improve human adaptation to nature, how substance use and abuse may act as a substitute for more serious deviance and even crime in a society, and how substance users may serve their group, culture, and historical era as messengers of critical issues or innovators of alternative lifestyles. At the concrete level, the functionalist perspective studies substance intake, substance users, and substance use in respective relation to the human body, individual groupings, and the sociocultural system. In specifying how the former contributes to the latter in various functional aspects, it examines and evaluates not only functions or positive effects, such as pain alleviation, symptom management, stress control, socializing, exchange, trade activities, service provision, and job creation, but also dysfunctions or negative consequences, such as dependency, withdrawal syndrome, social vice, crime, black market, wasting of social resources, and drain on taxpayers' money.

The rational choice perspective centers on human rationality in its effort to understand substance, substance use, and substance users. It examines why a substance is adopted for use, why certain substance use is regulated pertaining to age, gender, or occasion, and how individuals make their choice about use or nonuse, all under the premise of human rationality. While it primarily follows rationality in its normal functioning, the rational choice perspective logically points to irrationality for critical inquiry. For instance, can users make normally rational choices under the influence of drugs? Are there clouded reasoning, twisted rationality, or impaired judgment in the context of addiction? The rational choice perspective also investigates what range of rationality or irrationality a society may exhibit in its reaction to substance use and abuse as a social problem.

The social control perspective focuses on the unnecessary and harmful nature of substance use. It assumes that substance use is an unnatural, irrational, abnormal, and deviant behavior. People normally do not use substance. A few who use substance begin with a loosening or a lack of proper restraints in family, school, work, or other social settings. Once they use substance, they may experience a further loss of control in their life. To prevent substance use is to institute and strengthen proper social control measures. To intervene in substance abuse is to restore order and to gain control. Theoretically, the social control perspective analyzes social control in two dimensions: attachment and regulation. Attachment refers to ties and connections one forges with his or her family, groups, community, and society. Regulations include moral advice and legal guidance one receives from his or her parents, teachers, employers, and governing authorities. Social control problems arise when attachment or regulation becomes either insufficient or excessive.

The social disorganization perspective follows substance users to their living environment. On the one hand, it examines why individuals move from one environment to another, how they struggle to adjust to a new environment, and how they are lured or forced into substance use, deviance, or criminal activity in the face of difficulty from the new environment or due to their individual misadjustment. On the other hand, it studies how a particular environment changes from generation to generation, how drastic change in a specific environment causes stress, disillusion, and disorder among individuals who live in it, and why substance use, deviance, crime, and other social problems tend to increase in a time when or in a place where change occurs abruptly. In contemporary society, substance use and abuse are bound to be prevalent and high as individuals are constantly bombarded with social and market changes fueled by scientific discoveries and technological innovations.

The social learning perspective focuses on the behavioral dimension of substance use. It explores how substance use is acquired as a human behavior. Specifically, it studies what social situations are defined as favorable to, what motivations and rationalizations are required for, and what skills and techniques are involved in substance use. It also examines how the consequence of substance use feeds back on the process of learning and whether substance use can be unlearned through messages, groupings, and sources of influence unfavorable to violations of social norms. In approaching substance users as learners, for example, the social learning perspective points out that substance users are essentially influenced by whom they are associated with, whom they become identified with, what moral messages they are exposed to, what technical complexities they are taught with, what rewards they are given, what penalties they face, and what subculture they are thrown into in the process of learning and sustaining substance use. With proper changes in internal motivation and external pressure, users may learn to exit from or unlearn substance use by modes, through stages, under contingencies, and in contexts similar to those of learning.

The social reaction perspective capitalizes on the interactive nature of the three-way relations among substance users (actor), substance use (act), and societal responses (audience). It attempts to describe and explicate how one shapes and is shaped by another in a cyclical sequence involving all three variables. Beginning with substance use, for example, the social reaction perspective explores and explains why it is initiated, pursued, and cherished or avoided, resisted, and hated by actual and prospective users; why it is prompted, sanctified, and perpetuated or prohibited, stigmatized, and eliminated by society; and most essentially, how societal reactions implicitly and explicitly influence the way users see and behave themselves, the way they view and continue their substance use, and the way they perceive and approach life, work, society, and the whole world. Drawing upon the social reaction perspective, agents in social control should not spend all their time and energy on labeling substances, chasing substance users, and blaming a morally decaying generation or society for rampant substance use and abuse. They should instead keep some time and space to reflect upon the way they set up rules, educate the young, define deviance and crimes, approach substance use, and treat substance users. In some situations, the best way to react to substance use is to take no action at all. In some situations, the less action taken, the better it is for substance use and users. But under all circumstances, users and uses themselves should first be given their full respective force in correcting, healing, or adjusting a temporarily problematic situation before any social reaction ever takes place.

Finally, the subculture perspective focuses on the inner workings of substance user groups and groupings. It examines what beliefs, values, norms, and rituals users develop and follow in preserving and sustaining their substance use. It inspects what props, tools, aids, and equipment users innovate and employ in preparing substances for use, in administering substances, or in sanctifying use itself. It explores why users come together and what keeps them in solidarity with each other in the process of use, in the aftermath of abuse, and in reaction to pressure from the outside. Noting that the substance subculture exists in a crowd of other subcultures, the subculture perspective examines substance-relevant subcultures, such as the youth subculture, prostitute subculture, gang subculture, and deviant subculture, to see how each of them relates to substance use as cause, collateral occurrence, or consequence. Recognizing that the substance subculture is part of the general culture, the subculture perspective studies how the substance subculture draws spiritual inspiration and material supplies from the general culture, and how it contributes special symbols, meanings, artifacts, and other residues to the general culture. More subtly, the subculture perspective points out that the substance subculture itself may be a victim of the general failure or crisis in modern and postmodern culture although it is often singled out, along with criminal and deviant subcultures, for moral condemnation and legal attacks by the larger society.

This is the first book to systematically apply sociological perspectives to substance use and abuse. In drawing upon major sociological concepts and theories, I attempt to show that established sociological perspectives can be comprehensively tested in the practical field of substance use and abuse for their validity and utility. In developing theoretical explanations for substance, substance use, and substance users, I want to demonstrate that the established field of substance use and abuse can be insightfully enlightened with major theoretical perspectives from sociology.

—1—

The Anomie Perspective

Society is not a flat collection of equally resourceful and fortunate individuals. It is constructed in a complex hierarchy where people are discriminatively positioned with differential access to power, status, capital, and opportunities. In some areas, people are so deprived of legitimate resources that they take socially disapproved means as their sensible ways of survival. During some periods of time, people are so mercilessly denied opportunities by both conventional and unconventional worlds that they turn to substance use as their ultimate retreat from productive life. Among some social classes of people, mainstream norms and values seem to be so remote and irrelevant that subcultural and unconventional rules and beliefs become guiding principles in daily behavior.

The anomie perspective looks at substance use as resource, opportunity, or means in people's reaction to their specific social structural conditions. As resource, substance may be used to achieve material success. Substance use may be initiated and sustained to gain social status. As opportunity, substance may be used to excuse failure in the life struggle. Substance use may be attempted to escape from active social functioning. As means, substance may be touted as a coping mechanism. Substance use may be instituted as a routine defense against disappointment, frustration, and strain in personal experience with society.

SOURCES OF INSPIRATION

The concept of anomie was first coined by Emile Durkheim to denote a state of normlessness. According to Durkheim, human beings are born with "inextinguishable thirst" and have an insatiable and bottomless abyss of capacity for desires and feelings. In order for people to live together in groups and society, norms and moral authorities need to be developed and established to keep individual aspirations, passions, and desires in check.

In traditional society or society characterized by what Durkheim called mechanical solidarity, people live in closely knit communities. They attend the same church, go to the same marketplace, and share strongly in the same collective conscience. Children grow up in direct contact with parents, relatives, and neighbors. People receive concrete and clear directions and guidance in their everyday thoughts and behaviors. Anomie rarely occurs. When it does, it only appears as a random, accidental, temporal, isolated, or group-specific event. For example, unrelated individuals commit anomic suicide when they are thrown into normative confusion and moral ambivalence by some highly unexpected fortunes or misfortunes in life, such as a sudden rise or fall in personal wealth or status.

In contemporary society or society featuring organic solidarity, people live in increasing distance from one another as well as from the state. "Religion has lost most of its power. And government, instead of regulating economic life, has become its tool and servant. . . . Industry, instead of being still regarded as a means to an end transcending itself, has become the supreme end of individuals and societies alike. Thereupon the appetites thus excited have become freed of any limiting authority" (Durkheim 1952: 255). Although development of intermediate structures or secondary groupings, such as unions, occupational organizations, professional associations, and interest clubs, may provide a functional alternative to the old loyalties generated by religion, regionalism, and kinship, anomie is likely to remain a chronic social problem in the modern and postmodern world. Individuals, caught in a normative vacuum between the remote state and unscrupulous individualism, are likely to commit anomic deviance or offense, or fall victim of anomic suicide.

Anomie also takes place discretely in history when society switches from mechanical to organic solidarities. As the old value system breaks down and new moral doctrines scramble to emerge, people experience disruption, contradiction, loss of direction, and frustration in their thoughts and acts. It is also during the period of transition that instinctually based human greed is unleashed, pushing people into the shameless pursuit of their unlimited aspirations. Anomie, in this historically characteristic show-off, signifies not only confusion, helplessness, and strain, but also ambition, manipulation, and pleasure on the part of individuals.

A major turning point in the development of anomie theory appears in Robert Merton's 1938 essay "Social Structure and Anomie." Drawing upon the social experience of twentieth-century America, Merton redefined anomie as the structured disparity between promises of achievable prosperity and real-life opportunities to realize those promises. Like Durkheim, Merton examined unfulfilled aspirations to see how they affect people's mind and behavior. Unlike Durkheim, Merton focused on the socially structured disjuncture between culturally inspired aspirations and socially approved means for goal attainment, rather than normative confusion and chaos, to develop explanations for individual modes of adaptation.

In the United States, the majority of the population, including newcomers, seem to be identified with the mainstream middle-class values about the American dream. Through family, school, community, mass media, and other socialization agents, people are educated to believe that America is a fair and just society. Anyone who follows the rules, works hard, and is smart will be able to achieve material success and realize his or her American dream. The reality is, however, that social resources and opportunities necessary for material success are unequally and unevenly distributed across American society. Some are powerful, rich, and knowledgeable. Some are powerless, poor, and deprived of cultural capital. Some are born into the abundance of wealth and have ready access to a wide variety of opportunities. Some grow up in impoverished, gang-controlled, and violence-inflicted communities, and have to struggle hard in every step of their lives. While most people manage to live a conforming life in response to their specific social position, some individuals opt for nonconformist modes of adaptation in their reaction to blocked opportunities. There are innovators who adhere to culturally inspired goals but turn to socially illegitimate means to attain their goals. For example, inner-city gangs market drugs to achieve their economic prosperity. There are ritualists who play by the rules but do not care about success or personal advancement. For example, some corporate or governmental bureaucrats give up their hope for further upward mobility and desire only to get through their days until retirement. There are retreatists who abandon both cultural goals and legitimate means to retreat from active and productive social life. In Merton's list, they include "psychotics, artists, pariahs, outcasts, vagrants, tramps, chronic drunkards, and drug addicts" (1957: 153). Finally, there are rebels who formulate new standards and create new channels of opportunity to replace existing goals and means. For example, communist revolutionaries educate and organize proletarians in an attempt to create a society of equity and justice in place of capitalism.

Merton's general theory of deviance seems to imply that deviation is a choice for those who experience strain as they strive for success in the legitimate world. According to Richard Cloward and Lloyd Ohlin, however, opportunities for survival and success in the illegitimate world are not automatically, readily, and equally available and accessible either, to everyone who seeks them. Depending upon their specific living environment, youths who experience blocked opportunities in conventional society will engage in different activities, form different groups, and develop different modes of adaptation to life. In an environment dominated by organized for-profit criminal groups, alienated youths may serve their apprenticeship with professional criminals. They join crime-oriented gangs. They learn skills and disciplines. They aim to make a profit, keep a reputation, and earn a living from crime and deviance for themselves as well as for their devoted group. In an environment where adult criminals are largely unskilled, unsuccessful, and disorganized, youths are left with no role model, no live example, no technical teaching, and no organizational assistance for material success through illegitimate means. "Deprived not only of conventional opportunity but also criminal routes to 'big money'" (Cloward and Ohlin 1960: 180), youths form conflict-oriented gangs and engage in fighting and violence to vent anger, to cope with frustration, or to achieve status in the eyes of peers. Finally, in an environment clouded by an overwhelming sentiment of failure, despair, and normlessness, youths may withdraw from active and productive life in both conventional and deviant worlds. They take refuge in retreatist-oriented gangs. They center their attention and activity on the consumption of substances. They are only concerned with physical and emotional "highs." The last adaptation features what Cloward and Ohlin characterize as double failures who fail in both legitimate and illegitimate approaches to material success and social status.

Emphasis on group rather than individual responses to blocked opportunities is also reflected in Albert Cohen's work on delinquent boys. According to Cohen (1955), lower-class boys want to achieve success and higher social status just as much as their middle- and upper-class counterparts. Facing an unpromising social environment, however, lower-class boys divide into three groups in their response to the dominant middle-class value system. In college-boy response, they defer gratification, go to school, take up an occupational career, and attempt to conform to all other middle-class expectations. In corner-boy response, they give up competing with middle-class society and retreat to their specific lower-class subculture for some doses of self-perceived peace and comfort. Truancy, smoking, alcohol consumption, and drug use are common activities taken by corner boys. Finally in delinquent-boy response, youth act out in open defiance to middle-class values. They intentionally or unintentionally engage in behaviors deemed delinquent, malicious, or antisocial by the mainstream society.

Building upon his research on delinquency and the culture of gangs, Cohen went on to expand the anomie theory as a whole. Through his contribution, the anomie theory no longer looks atomistic and individualistic, as it first appears in Merton's formulation. Reference groups and social interactions are included in and related to the selection of adaptational alternatives by persons confronted with the strain of anomie. Deviant adaptation no longer seems to be discrete and discontinuous. It unfolds itself in a gradual, step-by-step process in which people shape and reshape behavior in response to their changing environment. Criminal deviance no longer appears to be practical and utilitarian only. It can become malicious, destructive, and harmful, not only by consequence, but also in terms of intentionality (Cohen 1965).

Upon the inspirations of the anomie perspective, sociologists and other disciplinary scholars pursue serious studies in drug abuse (Lindesmith and Simon 1964; Lewis 1970; Glaser, Lander, and Abbott 1971), suicide (Henry and Short 1954; Gibbs and Martin 1964; Maris 1969), and juvenile delinquency (Hirschi 1969; Freese 1973; Elliot and Voss 1974; Empey 1982; Triplett and Jarjoura 1997; Hoffmann and Su 1997). In substance use and abuse research, early studies center on the general assumption that drug users drop out into the retreatist subculture after an unsuccessful exploration of both legitimate and illegitimate avenues of goal attainment. Instead of supporting the assumption, empirical data indicate that initial choice of drugs is determined more by drug availability than by individual reaction to strain. Furthermore, as drugs are expensive and not easy to obtain, users have to work hard within the structures of both conventional and criminal worlds should they persist in their use habit.

Recently, some studies attempt to address the neglect of everyday stress by classic anomie theories. In a special issue on stress and substance use by *Substance Use and Misuse,* a number of researchers explore the fluctuations or temporal patterns of alcohol and substance use in relation to stress (Hoffmann 2000). Structural strain experienced by particular groups is beginning to gain attention. Scheier and Botvin (1996) find that minority youth engage in substance use, sensation-seeking, and unsafe behavior because they face sociopolitical and economic setbacks in addition to normal adolescent transition pressures. Hagedorn (1997) emphatically characterizes gang drug dealing as the innovative response of young minority males to blocked opportunity, rather than participation in a deviant, oppositional culture. Garcia (1999) argues that children who are subjected to racism; sexism; physical and mental abuse; inferior, dangerous schools; and abandonment to foster care from birth are doomed to lives of hopelessness, deviance, and drug use. Sharp, Terling-Watt, Atkins, Gilliam, and Sanders (2001) note that negative affective states, such as anger and depression, intervene in the relationship between strain variables and some prototypically female types of deviant behavior, including purging, bulimia, and substance use. Interest in the large environment and general social process continues. Zimny (2000) examines alcoholism and morality in Poland and eastern Europe, with reference to Russia. He senses a clear escapist reaction through alcohol and substance abuse by people who share exacerbated feelings of tension, alienation, despair, and uncertainty amid unemployment, currency devaluation, food shortages, and general social malaise.

THEORETICAL FRAMEWORK

The anomie perspective focuses on the disparity between individual aspirations and social resources in its quest for understanding of substance use and abuse. It is unique in the sense that individual attitudes and behaviors are examined against social structure and environmental conditions.

Definition

Anomie refers to both normlessness, as depicted by Durkheim, and strain, as portrayed by Merton. The connection in the two dimensions of the concept is twofold. On the one hand, problems in cultural assimilation and socialization cause moral confusion and normative extremism. Moral confusion makes individuals lose their sense of reality. At one extreme, they feel they are supermen or superwomen, they are above normal social rules, and they can do whatever they dream, desire, or want. At another extreme, they lament they are dwarfs, handicapped, or slaves of reality, they are restrained by every single social regulation, and they cannot reach even the simplest goal they set for themselves. Both extremes can lead to alienation and strain, creating either individual inclinations or social conditions for substance use and abuse.

On the other hand, failure, frustration, and strain experienced from social endeavors raise questions about self-expectation, ability, control, and image as well as social fairness, justice, legitimacy, and rationality. Moral unsureness, contradictions, and confusions ensue. In polarized reactions, individuals either harshly blame themselves to the degree of self-shame or critically charge society, even in the form of reversal, rebellion, or withdrawal. For example, they give up diligence, frugality, and conformity when they see none of those virtues works to their advantage. Substance use and other deviant behavior may arise amid moral dilemma or as part of individual reaction to social reality.

The anomie perspective follows anomie in both of its dimensions to study how substance use figures in as resource, opportunity, or means in the whole social-individual dynamic. Specifically, it examines how strain and moral undecidedness or loosening in normative control feed back on each other to make substance dealing, use, and addiction an attractive or acceptable reaction to life and reality.

Theoretical Image

Society is a resource, power, and status-differential structure. People are situated in different positions in the social hierarchy. Some lead. Some follow. Some live in affluence. Some fall under poverty. Some enjoy. Some suffer. Strain, uncertainty, and confusion, like joy, sureness, and clearness, are part of life and social dynamics.

Substance enters the picture of life as seduction, temptation, aid, companion, or scapegoat. People are seduced by some substances when they experience weak or loosening moral guidance from society. People are not able to resist the temptation of a substance and its mystified effects when they feel ambivalent and undecided about their approach to the substance because of a lack of knowledge. People turn to some substances for relief and comfort when they suffer from pain and stress in their life struggle. People use drugs to kill time, to feel at ease with themselves, or to beat loneliness in their temporary or permanent escape from active social life. Finally, people may symbolically take drugs as scapegoats for their personal anger, anxiety, stress, or failure although they themselves eventually bear the harm of the drugs. For example, one drinks alcohol, dumps it on the floor, and shatters the bottle as if alcohol is the thing to blame for his or her ill feelings at the moment.

Substance use takes place amid social strain and moral decline. Under strain, substance use is a coping mechanism, excuse, escape, defense, or rescuer. As a coping mechanism, it consumes frustration, channels anxiety, alleviates pain, and hopefully brings back peace and balance. For example, one feels "use of coffee helps me through the most stressful part of the task" or "use of alcohol gives me the courage to face creditors so that I can rebuild my failed business." As an excuse, substance use provides one with a publicly perceivable reason or explanation for why he or she drops out of social competition: "I have long had this use habit. It is now getting worse and worse. For the sake of the position I hold, I'd better leave." As an escape, substance use, abuse, and addiction pave the way to exit active social life. As a defense, substance use serves to protect one's self-image: "I have talents and potentials. I would have been a sure winner had I not been victimized by the evil effect of the substance." Substance use may also appear as a rescuer. For instance, youth who experience status frustration in mainstream social endeavors drink alcohol, smoke cigarettes and cigars, or use hard drugs to gain status among their peers as well as to prove their maturity, manhood, or womanhood in the eyes of adults. A substituted achievement in status through use of substance may indeed keep one from drifting into serious deviance in the aftermath of strain. Successful drug dealing directly makes up for any disadvantage, loss, or failure one experiences in the conventional world.

During moral decline, substance use increases when general beliefs, norms, and laws regarding substance and substance use become ambiguous, questionable, and ineffective. People ignore the law because it is controversial, incompatible with public perception, or unenforceable. Law enforcement agents are sympathetic to rule breakers and reluctant to deliver prescribed punishments when they see flaws and unreasonableness in the law. For example, drug laws do not always generate the same level of attention, respect, and enthusiasm as criminal laws from both the general public and the criminal justice system. At the individual level, substance use increases when people experience confusion and contradiction in their personal value, knowledge, and action systems. Confusion and contradiction occur when individuals change from one location to another; undergo an unexpected mobility in job or social status; hear different stories or interpretations regarding the benefit, legality, or moral appropriateness of substance use; or receive conflicting social treatments in their encounter with a substance.

Substance users are not just consumers of a substance. They are opportunists, drifters, sufferers, escapists, or double-failure retreatists, or the stressed, the confused, the weak-willed, or the lost. Opportunity users include those who take a substance to gain group-based status, who use and deal drugs for profit, and who use a substance because of loopholes in the law, loosening in law enforcement, change in social order, or general social chaos. Drifting users are those who do not have their own definite attitudes about substance and use a substance when a lot of people use it in a socially anomic situation. Suffering users turn to substances for help and relief as they struggle to manage the pressure they face in work and life. Escaping users engage in substance use to temporarily divert attention, to dispel fear, to hide their real feelings, or to avoid reality. Double-failure retreatists are those who withdraw from active life into drug addiction and dependency after failures in both the conventional and unconventional worlds. As a whole, substance users can all be considered as the stressed, the confused, the weak-willed, or the lost because they are not able to develop a clear personal value system about substance and substance use, and stand firmly with it, even in the strong current of unfavorable social influence.

Across society, groups that are discriminated against, repressed, exploited, isolated, or marginalized by or from the authority or mainstream are more likely to experience problems in cultural adjustment, blocked opportunities, economic deprivation, status frustration, and social stress. Members of those groups may hence engage more in substance use and abuse. Among different societies in the world, poor countries, nations under war and social unrest, states with a weak government or conflicting ideology, and regions in social transformation are more likely to fall into economic depression, political disorderliness, moral confusion, cultural chaos, and general social anarchy. Populations in those societies may therefore be more vulnerable to substance misuse and dependency. In

Western societies, although industrialization and urbanization are followed by considerable material affluence and social development, the division between haves and have-nots continuously generates and fuels conflict, confrontation, and tension across the populace. Individuals who socialize and resocialize through standardized education and synchronized mass media share to a large degree their beliefs, values, and norms about social order, social justice, and individual responsibility as well as their dreams, desires, and expectations toward the future, scientific discovery, technological innovation, and human progress. However, since they are born into dramatically different familial, communal, and social backgrounds, individuals face enormously different social challenges and opportunities in their work and life. Stress has become part of the Western psychosyndrome. Substance use, misuse, abuse, addiction, and dependency are now characteristic phenomena in Western contexts, not only by prevalence, but also in terms of persistence.

Throughout history, periods of revolution, reform, war, internal strife, and civil disturbance are more likely to foster moral ambivalence, ideological extremism, and behavioral confrontations. Times of drought, floods, famine, epidemics, and other natural disasters are more likely to feature fear, stress, and hopelessness. Substance use and abuse may thus expand widely across a population and rise sharply to an alarmingly high level. In the contemporary era, since people are constantly exposed to and inspired by different material achievements and lifestyles through advanced means of communication and transportation, they consistently wrestle with both internal strain and external tension between motivation and constraint, between expectation and outcome, and between dream and reality. People feel lucky when they succeed. They feel unlucky when they fail. Sentiments surrounding luck and fortune feed and fuel misconceptions about rules and norms in society. Easily, people take on a belief, follow a crowd, and chase a vogue. Frequently, they give up their hope, dump their plan, and abandon their effort. The general attitude of cynicism and the symptomatic feeling of uncertainty may provide the ultimate background why substance use and abuse remain high and widespread in the modern and postmodern era.

Theoretical Components

The anomie perspective places substance users under specific social structural conditions individuals face in their lives. Of primary importance to the perspective are four theoretical components.

Anomie: Confusion versus Strain

Anomie takes place either in the form of normlessness, lack of direction, and confusion, or in the form of frustration, disappointment, and strain. Substance use in reaction to anomie can have different features, meanings, and outcomes under those two forms and their respective subforms.

Moral confusion occurs in various circumstances. The most common situations include: overregulation, lack of regulation, conflicting regulation, and change in regulation. First, regulation is not limited to rules, laws, and law enforcement. It may involve knowledge, political climate, and public attitude. In the case of overregulation, individuals feel confused when they see little justice or no rationality in various social policies or practices in comparison to what they themselves perceive in their commonsense value system. For example, some adults feel they do a twenty-year-old youth a favor when they buy him or her cigarettes or alcohol because they see it absurd to disallow anyone over eighteen to drink or smoke. Lack of regulation is the opposite. In some typical scenarios, underage children pick up and smoke cigarette butts in the street. Low-quality or contaminated alcohol products flood the market. Addictive medications flow from hospitals to street corners. People fall under confusion and ambivalence because they wonder if social order will ever reign and human decency will ever prevail amid chaos, indulgence, and lack of spirituality. Conflicting regulation may involve situations where laws governing production, distribution, and consumption of a substance are inconsistent, where public reports regarding the harms or benefits of a substance are contradictory, and where social perception about the right and morality of individuals in substance use becomes erratic. For instance, people increase consumption, decrease use, switch from one form to another, or stop using it altogether out of confusion about conflicting scientific findings about the health effects of alcohol. Finally, change of regulation includes not only changes in social environment, such as repeal of law, enactment of law, strengthening law enforcement, and restricting social tolerance, but also changes in personal circumstance, such as migration, immigration, and job relocation. In history, sudden and dramatic changes in substance use follow the communist revolution as well as several prohibition crusades against alcohol in some parts of the world. At the individual level, rural migrants can be thrown out of balance when they see alcohol, cigarettes, coffee, tea, and other substances are so readily available in so many varieties through so many stores or channels across the city. So can immigrants from Third-World to First-World countries. Confusion, along with surprise and curiosity, can become an ever-powerful force for some newcomers to renew, intensify, and sustain their past interest in substance use.

Strain, as experienced by individuals in their social environment, does not always fully objectify itself in the modes of deviant adaptations. Conformists, in their effort to conform, may have to experience far more strain, in terms of variety, severity, and amount, than nonconformists who channel their strain through open deviations. Conformity strain ranges from status strain, success strain, and role strain, to nonfault strain. Status strain stems from a particular status, such as age, gender, race, ethnicity, celebrity, or fitness model, one is ascribed or achieves through his or her own effort. For example, an overage person colors his or her gray hair to look young. An actress takes dietary supplements or some hormones to stay slim or to keep her breasts in shape under the limelight. Success strain centers around work, performance, and achievement records. Artists take exotic drugs to enhance their creative instincts. Working professionals consume coffee and cigarettes to stay alert on challenging tasks. Athletes follow their coach or doctor's advice on diet and medications to ensure that they perform to their ultimate capability while remaining negative on standard tests in major competitions. Role strain derives from specific roles one has to play in work and life. For example, one seeks relief from alcohol when he or she feels stressed to handle a multitude of roles or to fit into one particular role. Nonfault strain relates to social expectations as well as individual wishes that one looks positive, knows what is right, behaves appropriately, and never misconducts him- or herself, from private bedroom to public places. Staying on track, individuals may have to use cosmetic materials, fragrances, medicines, and even drugs as their indispensable aids. Finally, for those who are forced into deviant adaptations, strain itself does not automatically dissipate into nonexistence. It still follows and haunts them as a process in life. The difference between conformists and nonconformists in their respective processual experience with strain is: the former contain strain by internal forces and the latter reveal it through external activities, with or without aid from substances in both cases.

Substance and Substance Use: Resource, Opportunity, and/or Means

Substance use in reaction to anomie runs a full gamut of variability in terms of intentionality, mood, act, and outcome. Users may intentionally seek assistance from substance use or unwillingly fall a victim of a substance in the weakest moment of their free will. They may feel positive or negative about use because they are in or out of control of the effect of a substance. They may turn things around or subject themselves to the power of addiction or the vicissitudes of circumstance. Anomie may therefore escalate, exacerbate, abate, dissipate, or disappear in the aftermath of substance use.

From a utilitarian point of view, however, substance and substance use can be focally seen as resource, opportunity, and/or means in response to anomie. Resource refers to the potential and practical utility of substance, substance use, and substance dealing in improving the prospect of material success and enhancing status for those who experience blocked mobility and status frustration. Youths who are no longer cared for or protected by their parents as children and who are not yet given proper rights or responsibilities as adults may find substance and substance use a resource to gain and secure status in the eyes of peers. In the beginning, they experiment with a substance often out of confusion or due to a lack of knowledge about the benefit, legality, or morality of its use. But when they feel like or are cheered as an adult by smoking, drinking, or doing drugs, they will actively take advantage of substance and substance use as a resource in their characteristic period of status frustration: "I handle it as well as any adult"; "He looks as cool and mature as any adult when he smokes"; and "He is as brave and adventurous as any adult when he takes that real stuff!" Similarly, an adolescent first sells or transports a packet of drugs because he or she does not know much about conventional efforts for monetary reward. He or she will drop out of school, join a drug-dealing ring, and take drug dealing as a professional undertaking and a way of material success when he or she realizes how difficult it would be to achieve the same level of wealth through conventional endeavor. People in the community will also change their attitude about the adolescent: "He or she is never caught by the police"; "He or she brings home a lot of money"; "He or she indeed is smart and has a talent, although he or she does poorly in school and seems to have no hope for success in any conceivable mainstream engagement"; and "Dealing drugs seems to be what he or she is best at doing."

Opportunity centers around the scapegoat function substance and substance use may serve for some strained individuals. They cite a substance and its possible effect in their explanation for job dereliction, neglect of duty, delay in schedule, or inadequate performance if they use the substance regularly. They blame the abundance of supply, the popularity of use, or the stress of life when they tell stories about why they start using substances. They refer to their preoccupation with drugs, drug supply, drug addiction, side effects, and treatment when they quit a job, escape their family, and withdraw from other social responsibilities. Substance and substance use thus become not only a shield against internal feelings of incompetency, inadequacy, or guilt, but also an excuse from external pressures for success and responsible role playing. Some typical opportunistic reasoning includes: "There is nothing wrong with me"; "It's just that substance that messes up everything"; "Addiction is a disease"; "Anybody can contract that disease"; "You can't do anything when you are addicted"; and "It's OK to stay in drug addiction, away from stress and normal social functioning."

Means focuses on the effects of substance and substance use in helping people manage stress, cope with difficult situations, and keep things under control. Using substance as a means toward control lies in public belief, historical practice, and social fashion. In a culture oriented to the power of spirit, people may not call upon any substance in their dealings with the outside world, whereas in a culture built upon materials, people may explore every possible substance for answers and solutions to any problems they face in life. For example, they take pain killers when they feel pain in some parts of their body. They swallow sleeping pills when they have difficulty falling asleep. They drink spirit when they feel cold or are afraid. They turn to fitness medications if they want to lose or gain weight. They drink tea or coffee when they wake up for work. Or they consume drugs just to make some statements. As far as anomie is concerned, there are specific pressures on appearance, performance, and general social functionality. People may have to use, with the danger of misuse and abuse, a variety of substances to look young, look beautiful, or just fit in everyday life; to stay competitive, productive, or just competent on the job; and to remain positive, respectful, or just attentive in social occasions.

Anomie and Substance Use: Individual Adjustment

Moral confusion and strain are part of individual feelings and experiences. Substance use is an individual act. No matter how the social environment is inducive or facilitative in the occurrence or sustenance of anomie and substance use, it is individuals who make critical decisions about what to do in response to particular social situations.

With respect to anomie, individuals can stick to their past experiences, draw upon some familiar rules, or play one simple game they know in a normless, rule-conflicting, norm-changing, or otherwise complex situation. They may remain calm and quiet, letting time take care of the matter. They may quickly burn and bury their past learning, embracing the new situation with a fresh mind and a nonassuming attitude. Confusion may occur now and then but will never materialize into a depressing mental condition. Similarly, individuals can diversify aspirations, lower goals and standards, or adjust frames of reference in their lives and professional pursuits. They may focus on patience and persistence, putting success into a long-term perspective. They may even dampen or dim their instincts about success, recasting life as just an endless striving toward peace. Anxiety, stress, and senses of tiredness or boredom may flash here and there but will never grow into a devastating feeling of despair.

Even when anomie takes hold, individuals can take a variety of actions, positive or negative, active or passive, to avoid substance and substance use as a way out or a way in. Substance and substance use become an option usually to those individuals who know about a substance and its effects, who have access to a substance and its dealers, who network with existing users, and who identify with various skills and motives of use. By closing out avenues to or nullifying conditions for substance and substance use, individuals may automatically opt for other choices in sight.

In the case of moral confusion, individuals may seek spiritual or religious conversions. In response to pressure for success, individuals may turn to inner forces rather than material stimulants or depressants for assistance. For example, one may engage in exercise to stay fit or practice Taiji or Qigong to rejuvenate him- or herself at work. Even a retreatist path does not necessarily entail or coincide with substance use and abuse. One may withdraw from secular life by becoming a monk or nun in a temple or just wander around in the street as a drug-free vagrant, homeless person, or beggar.

Anomie and Substance Use: Social Conditioning

Although individual adjustment makes a difference in the onset of anomie and substance use, social conditioning provides the ultimate background in which individual choice is made. What choices are available within a given social environment? What choice is favored by society?

As far as anomie is concerned, cultural, moral, and legal systems are not always developed and integrated to the ultimate standards of rationality and coherence. There are ambiguities, contradictions, loopholes, inconsistencies, and room for interpretation and deviation. Enforcement can be contaminated with personal biases and individual flavors. People naturally wonder if there is any justice when they see drastically different outcomes for similar acts committed by different individuals. Change in law, morality, and culture may come slowly, rapidly, regionally, globally, partially, or wholesale. People are often off guard when they are forced into various modes of adaptation. In an open society driven by market forces, the pace of life is inherently high. Materials flow from place to place. Science and technology change with every passing day. Information circulates instantly among the population. People can easily be lost in the strong current of a socially activated and fueled mobile lifestyle.

Aside from moral confusion, resources and opportunities are unequally distributed across the population. Some accumulate too much wealth, gain too much status, or wield too much power so that they feel they are above the social norm, they can do anything they want, they have to keep what they have, or they need to appear in elegance, generosity, nobleness, or whatever favorable image they perceive to be in the eyes of the public. Some are so poor, so low in status, or so powerless that they do not even know whether they have anything to eat for the next meal or anywhere to stay for the next day, whether they are any better than their master's favored pets, or whether they will be interrogated, beaten, or abused in the next hour. Some are born to wealth and are surrounded by opportunities. Some stay forever in poverty and social deprivation no matter how bright they are and how hard they try. Strain obviously is socially produced and reproduced. It impacts both the rich and the poor, the advantaged and the disadvantaged, the powerful and the powerless, albeit in totally different forms.

The connection from anomie to substance and substance use is also made in large part by social conditions. First, substance is differentially available to societies across the globe. Some are areas of production and supply. Some are corridors of trafficking and transport. Some are places of trade and exchange. Some are destinations of use and consumption. Second, substance use is differentially favored by cultures in the world. There are spiritually oriented cultures in which people are conditioned to rely upon the power of the mind to solve problems in morality and reality. There are material cultures in which people are spoiled to indulge in substance and substance use as ultimate means and ends in life. For a similar type of strain, one in a material culture may use drugs to cope while his or her counterpart in a spiritual culture may turn to seclusion, meditation, or conversion for answers or solutions. Third, substance and substance use grow into different patterns of selection by people in varying geographic locations. Alcohol abuse increases among Russians in their social transformations from communism to capitalism first because alcohol has been their default substance of coping or substance of choice for generations. Finally, individuals are born to different communities, social networks, and historical periods with different levels of knowledge and attitudes about and different accesses to substance, substance use, and drug dealing. One is able to turn to drug dealing for material success often because he or she is born to a family or neighborhood where he or she can take apprenticeship with an experienced dealer or can enter a well-established drug dealing ring or cartel.

Theoretical Applications

Focusing on the connection between anomie and substance use, a variety of abstract as well as concrete questions can be raised and investigated to broaden and deepen our understanding of the human mind and behavior.

First, are human beings inherently liable or vulnerable to substance use and abuse? Under normal conditions, human beings drink water, eat foods, or take medications so that they stay in the regular range of perception, feeling, performance, and functionality. They tend to use and abuse substances when they fall into moral confusion or strain. Does this mean that human beings are tamed slaves of control, peace, or order? As such, do they automatically or inevitably go astray in the form of substance abuse if they are not given proper guidance or when they are upset?

Second, are substance use and abuse natural and necessary conditions corresponding to anomie? In the mind of individuals, anomie is a mental state, a self-experience of disorientation, lack of direction, frustration, and anxiety. Does that mental state need a turbulent bodily condition as foundation, background, or companion? In other words, is substance used and abused to create and sustain a level of tension in the body comparable to the level of strain experienced in the mind?

Third, do substance use and abuse serve to correct or reverse the condition of anomie? In its correctional function, does a substance act on the body, bringing it to a prime or desirable level of energy, endurance, and productivity? Does it target the mind, calming it down, straightening it out, or lowering the level of fear, prohibition, or expectation it institutes upon itself? Or does it work on the synchrony between body and mind, reconciling one with another in the process of goal setting and task performance?

Fourth, do substance use and abuse confirm or reinforce a situation of confusion or strain? In confirmation, does substance use serve as a public statement about one's social condition? Does it make one aware that he or she has failed or is not able to handle the situation all on his or her own? By reinforcement, does substance give one the illusion that he can go back while in fact it pulls him further away from his intended goal? Does one fall gradually and deeply into substance dependency because one's initial experience with substance makes him feel that substance is beneficial and he can get away from substance use in both legal and psychological terms? Is it possible that confirmation serves one as a reality check to bring him or her back to the normal? Similarly, how probably does reinforcement hit one with a bottom situation from which he finds motivation to jump back to his previous life?

Finally, do substance and substance use just divert attention from anomie without any direct alleviating or reinforcing effects on it? Diversion occurs when one substitutes his or her moral confusion or strain with substance experience. In drunkenness, he or she no longer worries about directions in life or responsibilities at work. Under addiction, he can excuse himself from any moral dilemma and life endeavor. While diversion is a major theme under retreatism, does it figure temporarily in non-retreatist situations? Is the original moral confusion or strain just left unattended? Is any new confusion or strain produced when attention is shifted to substance use and abuse? Does substance use shift or dim attention to life-related strain?

Empirical Tests

The anomie perspective creates opportunities for empirical research. Test of the perspective with respect to its various specific propositions calls for use of different research designs and methods (Bailey 1994; Hagan 2000).

Case studies follow individual users to see if they fall into substance use and abuse because of normal confusion, stress in life, or a retreatist choice. Specific cases may help to illustrate various situations between anomie and substance use. For example, one starts using a substance in a legally or morally vague environment. He or she later enters into an environment of legal or moral clarity and definiteness. In the new environment, he or she faces pressure to quit the substance use. Would the pressure one experiences to quit serve as a strain to sustain one's use habit? Another example is: one uses a substance when he or she faces a temporal yet tremendous strain in life. He or she passes through the stressful episode later but becomes stuck to the substance as a habitual user. Would the chronic use he or she falls under serve as a positive or negative force in his or her future dealings with strain in life? Still another example is: one uses substances when he or she fails in endeavors in both the conventional and unconventional worlds. Would the substance use he or she is involved with serve as a health condition to withdraw into or from a retreatist lifestyle? Moral confusion, strain, and the idea of retreat come and go in life while substance use often stays as a habit or health condition. Individual cases can obviously supply valuable stories to fill various gaps and holes between abstractly conceptualized cause and effect in the anomie theory.

Historical analysis may be applied to study users, groups, and societies in their respective encounters with substances. Users, as they grow up from childhood through adolescence to adulthood, experience status change and frustration. They face social differentials and strain as they move upward or downward through job, power, wealth, and social class scales. Are there specific substances of use and abuse for children, adolescents, adults, and seniors, as well as for street beggars, blue-collar workers, white-collar professionals, and social elites? How do individuals deal with their evolving experiences with substances in response to change in age and social position? Groups may fall under anomic situations when they go through reorganization, expansion, or change in membership, solidarity, or collective sentiment. Patterns of substance use may emerge over time, showing increase or decrease between periods of anomie and normality in overall use or in the use of a particular substance. Similarly, societies progress amid confusion, conflict, contradiction, depression, turmoil, and general strain. In the time of anomie, the populace may indulge in or shun a particular substance. Overall use may rise or decline. Even substance itself can be studied in association with anomie. Based upon their unique correlations with anomie, some substances may be called substances of moral confusion, decline, or decay while others are dubbed substances of midlife crisis, professional stress, or social malaise.

Interview and survey are vital devices in uncovering how anomie and substance use relate to each other in specific details. Anomie, either in the form of moral confusion or in the form of strain, is what individuals experience in their inner world. Substance use is an individual act. Whether it affirms, alleviates, or exacerbates anomie can only be felt and described by users themselves. Interview targets selected users. It asks them in-depth questions so that specific details regarding anomic experience, substance encounter, and their interrelations can be documented in case studies as well as small-group researches. Survey covers a large population or a segment of the general population. By asking sampled subjects questions appropriate to their experience, researchers may be able to identify some common anomic symptoms and their corresponding substance use syndromes inherent in social life among the populace in a particular era. For example, under capitalist conditions, people have to spend years on education to enter the labor force. Jobs are not insured. People get on and off jobs through ruthless competition, selection, and elimination. Consumer goods are abundant in the market. People are lured to buy and consume through credit and by tides of fashion. Pressure to earn and spend money could throw a lot of people into acute or chronic anomie. The whole population may therefore float at a high level of propensity or risk for substance use and abuse.

Experimental studies can go one step further to examine biochemical balance or imbalance among subjects who suffer from acute or chronic strain. Insufficient or excessive presence of one or a few bodily chemicals may be linked to voluntary or involuntary intake of one or a cluster of substances in the form of regular use or abuse. Alternatively, substance dependency or addiction can be analyzed to see whether it weakens or strengthens human coping with stress, change, and challenge. Instead of opting for substance use because of his or her retreatist choice, it is possible that one falls into retreatism due to his or her substance use. In quasi-experimental design, various strategies and tactics can be used to determine whether anomie leads to substance use or vice versa or whether any other factors influence the correlation between anomie and substance. Suppose anomie has been positively identified as a cause of substance use. To test whether association influences the causal relationship from anomie to substance use, a sample of similarly positioned and stressed subjects can be selected and assigned to various association conditions, association with users, with stress counselors, with antidrug activists, or with the general public. Association with the general public may serve as a control condition to compare if and how any special association accelerates or decelerates the sequential change from stressful experience to substance use.

POLICY IMPLICATIONS

The anomie perspective delves into individual experience as well as social climate in its quest for understanding of substance use and abuse.

Users live in a social environment. They derive their individual experience from social interaction. They can modify and change their personal experience effectively only through social participation. Social agencies and agents therefore need to embrace both individuals and their social surroundings in dealing with substance and substance-related problems.

Public Health

Professionals and officials in public health can benefit from the anomie perspective at two major fronts. In prevention, they can design programs to educate the public about strain, life events, and social change. Stress is explored with respect to its source, type, nature, and coping strategies. Information about stress and relief is spread across the population. Long-term monitoring as well as short-term campaigns are implemented for groups at risk and with special needs. It is also important to ensure that people develop proper tolerance for the routinely high level of stress in contemporary life and be prepared to deal with different types of stresses through a diverse repertoire of approaches, with or without the aid of substance.

In intervention, health officials and professionals can focus on counseling, psychiatric diagnosis, trauma reaction, and mental illness treatment for service improvement and enhancement. Adjustments may be needed in attitude and behavior given the deep-rooted belief in medicine and long-established practice in mental health. First, stress is a serious health condition. It needs the same timely diagnosis and effective treatment as bodily diseases. Second, stress involves both physical and nonphysical dimensions. Diagnosis needs to be based upon full examination of all relevant factors in all possible aspects. Third, stress can be acute as well as chronic. It calls for both contingent and long-term care and attention. Finally, stress is a comprehensive medical problem. Treatment needs to go beyond medicine to incorporate emotional, spiritual, and social solutions. Medication and use of substance may prove useless if they are not integrated with psychological counseling, moral guidance, and social support. Also, use of medicine per se may lead to substance dependency and other health complications.

Obviously by preventing and treating stress and other anomic conditions, health professionals and officials may find themselves in a less stressful situation to deal with substance use and abuse.

Social Control

Social control ensures social order. It, however, may become a source of confusion, stress, and disorder as well.

Drawing from the anomie perspective, social control agencies and agents can reduce public confusion and frustration by making law clear, accessible, and understandable to the general population. A lot can be done given the fact that law is made by career politicians in the legislature, interpreted by judges in the court, and practiced or manipulated by lawyers between the system and their often fearful clients. In terms of content, there are unfair laws, discriminatory rules, and irrational regulations. They cause not only confusion but also agony and suffering for many people under their influence. As many nations are now still under authoritarian regime, one-party rule, or plain dictatorship and only the rich and powerful are seen to be elected to the legislature as people's representatives in democratic countries, it is obvious that there is a long way to go to a whole world of legal equity.

Enforcement is another important issue. Although many laws are written clearly and look fair in the book, they are not equally applied to people who come into contact with them. Some groups of people, types of acts, or geographic areas are targeted for intensified scrutiny while others have no official surveillance and monitoring. To ordinary people who perceive laws concretely in the hands of individual social control agents, unfair law enforcement causes most actual confusion, a sense of injustice, and a loss of hope. It is thus critical that social control agents overcome stereotyping and abandon profiling in terms of age, gender, race, ethnicity, education, income, or any other personal or socioeconomic variable. Instead, they should focus on acts, traits, and issues and always refrain from categorizing actors and jumping to conclusions about groups of people on the basis of individual acts or actors.

Still another important issue is how social control agents mediate between the state and people. Social control agencies and agents are windows of the state. The various ways they operate can give people different feelings and attitudes toward the government, the authority, and the whole social system. They may generate a public impression of a caring government, a protective authority, and a society of justice. They may also create a general image of a repressive government, a dominating authority, and a system of discrimination. As far as anomie is concerned, social control agents should first treat all common citizens with passion and respect. Second, they should put most of their emphasis on education and protection. Third, they should serve as role models for the general public. A caring social control force surrounding a gentle state can rally and unite people around major social causes. Public suspicion, resentment, and resistance can then be reduced and minimized. Social conflict, strain, and anomie can therefore be contained, diffused, and digested, which in the end may keep substance use and abuse under control.

Life and Community

Life is unpredictable. Confusion, disappointment, frustration, and failure are basic features in life. To manage unfavorable currents and events in the life course, one needs to first have a systematic view of himself or herself regarding his or her abilities, resources, social positions, ambitions, accomplishments, and goals. He or she then needs to develop basic understandings of essential contrasts in life: long-term versus short-term, part versus whole, past versus future, principle versus contingency, outside versus inside, personal versus social, and appearance versus substance. On the emotional dimension, he or she needs to be calm, strong, and self-confident, with proper preparation and tolerance for anomic incidence.

In the community, neighbors should treat each other as neighbors. They must overcome prejudice, avoid stereotyping, and embrace the diversity of lifestyle. The spirit of understanding and concern can be demonstrated on many specific events and encounters in everyday life. Sometimes, a minor gesture can convey a subtle yet important message, pulling a neighborhood from apathy, division, or tension to sharing, unity, or peace. Suppose a couple engage in an intense verbal argument within their house. Neighbors may call the police for intervention. They may stay silent and unresponsive as if nothing has happened. They may yell at them: "Could you guys please be quiet?" They may step in to offer help: they take one to a restaurant and the other to their private home for some cooling off or comfort. Different reactions from the community can have different impacts upon the couple. One possible scenario is that one of the couple runs to a local bar to get drunk and avoid embarrassment in front of his or her neighbors. Another example is: one turns on the light or walks in the neighborhood in the middle of the night because he or she is not able to fall asleep like everyone else. After complaints from other family members or the neighbors, he takes sleeping pills even though he knows he may someday become dependent upon the substance.

It is obvious that stress and anomie are not only generated but also disposed in life and the community. With proper attitudes and actions, one can manage anxieties, crises, emergencies, and various other problems in life well, without falling the victim of substance. By the spirit of mutual concern and support, neighbors can come together in the time of confusion, uncertainty, and difficulty, protecting their community from the dramatic onslaught of anomie and substance abuse.

Work and Organization

Work is a lifeline for most people in contemporary society. It is the ultimate yardstick to measure success, status, and the quality of life. Because of its critical importance, work is naturally a primary source of anxiety, stress, and anomie.

Drawing upon the anomie perspective, one first needs to do a reality check so he knows what he can realistically accomplish within his power. Second, one needs to overcome the temptation to dream high, target high, and achieve high. Failure to realize unrealistically ambitious goals can quickly turn to dispositions to retreat and problematic behavior. Third, one needs to avoid the tendency for comfort, complacency, and self-sufficiency. Regret over unrealized potentials and talents may also throw one out of balance. Fourth, one needs to develop a dynamic view of work, success, and failure. He or she is able to see the distinctions between one part of a job and the whole job, one type of work and a whole range of choices for work, and one-time failure and a whole career success. Finally, one needs to put work into proper perspective with marriage, family, and other life engagements. He or she understands work is not everything although it is one of the most important things.

Regarding work organizations, they first should establish a fair and equitable system for recruitment, evaluation, promotion, and discipline. Employees are not discriminated against in any way on the basis of their belief, race, gender, age, or personal background. Second, they should provide employees with clear guidance on their job duties, benefits, and upward mobility. New recruits are welcome with informative orientations. Job transferees are given specific retraining lessons. Open dialogues are maintained between supervisors and employees under their supervision. Third, employers should make a range of necessary information and counseling services available to their employees, from stress management, personal communications, and career development, to conflict resolution. Work generates stress. People experience ups and downs in their mood, ability, and performance. It is critical that employees be given assistance while they go through a difficult time. Finally, an employer should view itself as one of many employment organizations in the market that could or could not support an employee in his or her career endeavors. It is important that employment organizations serve as sources of inspiration and support rather than cages of containment or exploitation for career-bound professionals.

With proper approaches toward work by employees as well as proper approaches toward employees by employers, a critical amount of anomie can be taken away from the general population, making it less vulnerable for problem behaviors such as substance use and abuse.

In sum, the anomie perspective builds a bridge between social conditions and individual adjustments in its analysis of substance use and abuse. In examining social conditions, it reveals how moral confusion, anxiety, strain, and other anomic problems can be caused and sustained by flawed laws, biased policies, discriminative law enforcement, and in-equitable distributions of wealth, power, and opportunity. In inspecting individual adjustments, it shows how individuals may turn to substances as means, coping mechanisms, resources, and retreats in response to fail-ure, deprivation, discrimination, injustice, and general social pressure they experience from their social environment.

In light of the anomie perspective, one way to reduce substance use and abuse is to improve social conditions so that laws are made clear, acces-sible, and understandable to common citizens; laws and social norms are enforced fairly and equitably across the population; and, most important, social resources and opportunities are equally provided for all members of the society. On the individual side, people should understand that life is an open process, strain is part of life, and reactions to confusion and strain in life do not have to take a substance route. In fact, since strain comes and goes, substance use tends to stay as a habit, and substance use may interfere with individual ability to cope with stress, it is important that individuals develop proper tolerance for ambiguity, uncertainty, and anxiety; seek nonsubstance solutions for their personal problems; and par-ticipate in various social activities to bring positive change to their society.

The anomie perspective also notes that the fast pace and the perplex-ing complexity of work and life in contemporary society have created or added a new dimension or layer of confusion and strain among modern and postmodern individuals. Belief in science and reliance on medicine support a widely spread perception of and a deeply felt sentiment toward substance as the ultimate cure for ailments, diseases, and problems, from physical, psychological, emotional, and personal, to social. The combina-tion of a high level of anomie and an unquestionable trust in substance obviously explains why substance use and abuse exist and will continue to exist as an outstanding issue in the foreseeable future.

—2—

The Career Perspective

Substance abuse is a chronic condition. It involves a progression that usually moves through initiation, experimentation, habituation, dependence, problematic experience, assistance seeking, treatment, cessation, relapse, maturation, and abstinence. During this evolving process, users may experience various changes in physiological, psychological, personal, and social dimensions and take on different perspectives in work and life. Social reactions are usually fashioned accordingly through stages of individual change. For instance, prevention comes typically in the initial phases whereas treatment takes place when individuals develop serious symptoms of addiction.

The career perspective draws from the career dynamics theory in management and organizational studies. It parallels substance use and abuse to the employment career that features upward and downward mobility over the individual life span. The basic theme is that substance use and abuse invoke an evolutionary process that not only causes physiological, psychological, and personal changes across the users' life span, but also has economic and social impacts on their living environment.

SOURCES OF INSPIRATION

Career refers to "the evolving sequence of a person's work experiences over time" (Arthur, Hall, and Lawrence 1989: 8). As an important concept in management and organizational studies, it inspires various interests across scientific disciplines. In psychology, career is variably perceived as personality stability in adulthood, a vehicle for self-realization, a component of the individual life structure, and an individually mediated response to external role messages. From anthropology, economy, geography, history, and political science, to sociology, it is viewed respectively as status passages, a response to market forces, a response to geographic circumstances, a correlate of historical outcomes, the enactment of self-interest, and the unfolding of social roles (Arthur, Hall, and Lawrence 1989).

The concept of career was applied to the field of crime and deviance when Edwin Sutherland embarked on his study of the professional thief. According to Sutherland (1937), the professional thief makes crime a regular business undertaking and a way of life. He acquires specialized attitudes, knowledge, skills, and experiences, devotes his entire working time and energy to stealing, and organizes his life around his criminal pursuits. Career is applied in its original meaning as the professional thief takes stealing as his occupation and means of livelihood. The only difference is that he makes his career through an illegal rather than a conventional line of activity.

A relatively indirect use of career is found in Howard Becker's study of outsiders. Becker (1963) applied career to denote the measurable process by which outsiders develop and maintain their deviant role and status. On marijuana use in particular, he found that users are not just "lay" people. They need to learn how to get high, manage the feeling of high, gain access to supply, and build peer support networks. All these take time and effort, which makes marijuana use, or deviance in general, comparable to a professional career pursuit.

In substance use research, studies that build on the concept of career fall into four main categories: addiction career, natural history, pathway arguments, and lifestyle hypotheses. Addiction career is generalized from studies on hard drug use (Musto 1999). For narcotics, an addiction career includes experimentation, escalation, maintenance, change, recovery, and ex-addiction (Waldorf 1983). Addicts may alternate between addiction and nonaddiction throughout their career as measured by drug use and criminal involvement (Hanlon, Nurco, Kinlock, and Duszynski 1990). Cocaine addiction follows a similar career path, although change through stages takes different patterns. Escalation, for instance, can proceed in four modes: mild-moderate-severe, mild-severe, moderate-severe, and severe only (Khalsa, Paredes, and Anglin 1993).

Natural history describes drug use along with the natural process of growth, maturation, and aging. It attempts to pinpoint how substance use and abuse correlate with physiological, psychological, and social changes throughout the individual life course. The general observation is that substance use breaks out at youth, escalates during adolescence, stabilizes and matures throughout adulthood, and regresses in the senior stage. Specifically, some studies point out that substance use ceases around the age of thirty and no initiation into alcohol and cigarettes and hardly any initiation into illicit drugs occurs after that age (Chen and Kandel 1995). As far as treatment is concerned, some studies diversify the route of natural history from developmental change to spiritual conversion, environmental change, retirement, substitution, and drift into the mainstream (Waldorf 1983), whereas others explore conditional factors in the developmental change of maturing out or maturation (Anglin, Brecht, and Woodward 1986).

Pathway arguments attempt to portray the general path of progression or sequence for the use of different substances, licit or illicit, with or without specific reference to age, gender, or race. A typical pathway is that users begin with legal substances, such as alcohol and tobacco; they then proceed to marijuana; and they later progress to hard drugs, such as heroin and cocaine. An implicit assumption is that drug effects build up and mild substances serve as a gateway to the use of moderate drugs, which in turn pave the way for initiation to hard drugs. Two variables are apparently relevant to the drug use pathway. One is age: use of alcohol or tobacco often starts in early adolescence; marijuana arrives in the drug use scene around the mid-teens; and onset to hard drugs usually occurs in the late teens and early twenties (Kandel, Yamaguchi, and Chen 1992). The other variable is the drug era: a specific period of time when a particular drug becomes popular among some age or social groups or across the general population. According to a study of hard-drug users in New York, older crack users, who were born before the early 1950s and experienced both the heroin injection era (1963–1973) and the cocaine powder era (1975–1984), are more likely to follow a pathway that involves gateway drugs, intravenous drug use, cocaine snorting, and crack smoking (Golub and Johnson 1994). In contrast, younger crack users who were born between 1968 and 1972 are more likely to proceed directly from gateway drugs to crack smoking (Golub and Johnson 1994). Gateway drugs include both licit substances, such as alcohol and tobacco, and illicit drugs, such as marijuana.

Lifestyle hypotheses approach drug use as a lifestyle that emerges from an interacting network of influences, including conditions, choice, cognition, and change (Walters 1994). Conditions can be internal (heredity and temperament) or external (family and peers), positive (protective factors) or negative (risk factors). They do not cause drug use by themselves but may predispose users to drug use by affecting their life options. Choice is made by individuals from the life options established by their conditional parameters. Cognition refers to individuals' conscious efforts to rationalize decisions they have made in life. Although conditions, choice, and cognition steer people to particular lifestyles, change is possible when intervention is effectively directed to life influences in their natural sequence. For instance, interventions can be designed to assist drug users to manage life conditions, improve decision-making competence, and learn cognitive patterns in support of a drug-free lifestyle (Walters 1994).

A career perspective on substance use and abuse can, therefore, draw upon not only theoretical studies of employment career, deviance, and criminal behavior, but also various specific explanations of drug use and abuse derived from empirical research.

THEORETICAL FRAMEWORK

Substance use and abuse begin with four interrelated prerequisites: users, substance, time, and space. The career perspective, as it attempts to capture the process or the time dimension of substance use and abuse, has to look into user characteristics, the nature of substance, and the social context of use to find out how they fashion different paths of use career.

Definition

Substance use career refers to the evolving sequence of substance use and abuse over time. Specifically, it variably refers to the evolutionary path of a user's drug experience through life span, the general progression of a drug's use and abuse across the population, and the socially perceived or observed sequence of use and abuse among identified substances. Borrowed from the field of work and employment, career is nonetheless not used to legitimate drug use and abuse as a conventional domain of activity. Nor is it used to justify drug use and abuse as a sustainable lifestyle one can meaningfully carry on through his or her life. It is used just to capture the entrenched effect of substance use and abuse on human beings, their mind and body.

The career perspective builds on the concept of career and approaches substance use and abuse as a dynamic process that unfolds over time. In its uniqueness, it (a) emphasizes the changing character of drug use and drug users; (b) stresses the accumulative effect of use or nonuse episodes over a sequence of progression or regression; and (c) attends to the interaction of user characteristics, drug factors, and social influences through an evolutionary process. The career perspective serves a multitude of purposes: a theoretical model, a methodological device, and a policy guide. It holds various implications for public health, social control, community, and organizational reactions to the problem of substance use and abuse.

Theoretical Image

Drug use is not a static state. It is a changing condition. Change in drug use and abuse does not just feature a stochastic process. It takes place through progressive or regressive stages that reflect both the effect of accumulation and the interaction of various influences in the process of change. Most saliently, drug use and its evolutionary change make different career pathways behind drug users, drugs, and social environments or historical eras.

For drug users, a general use career pathway runs through nonuse, initiation, experimentation, escalation, habituation, problematic experiences, treatment, temporary abstinence, relapse, maturing out, retirement, and total abstinence. Individual variations, however, can occur in every possible combination due to user characteristics, drug effects, and social factors. For instance, death from drug overdose may occur right after escalation, concluding a drug use pathway without later career stages. Encounter with law enforcement may come during experimentation, making the socially problematic experience jump the path over escalation and habituation. A problematic experience in turn may either pull a user out of his or her premature use career or push him or her into dependent use over a career pathway.

With respect to user characteristics in particular, age overall can predict different career pathways. Whereas users at an older age may have already experienced a long drug use history, those of a younger age can be expected to make steady strides through the main stages of a use career. At a particular career stage, age may foretell users' possible progression or regression in drug use. Nonusers after thirty usually no longer experience any formal onset to drugs while those maturing out after sixty are likely to stay in abstinence for the rest of their life (Chen and Kandel 1995; Anglin, Brecht, and Woodward 1986). Race can influence use career through different drug preferences among ethnic groups. Compared to Caucasian powder cocaine users, who may closely follow the general career pathway, African American crack smokers may escalate their use after experimentation and, therefore, run into problematic experiences before habituation (Shaw, Hser, Anglin, and Boyle 1999). Socioeconomic status can make a difference on drug career as well. Economically advantaged users are usually able to protect and maintain their habit through naturally evolving career stages, whereas resources-stressed users can be interrupted frequently from their drug use career by lack of social support and law enforcement interventions. Moreover, user characteristics may work in various combinations with each other as well as with drug factors and social parameters, making different use configurations or histories out of the general career pathway.

Each drug may develop a general use pattern due to its chemical composition, pharmacological properties, and interaction processes with human biochemical and neuropsychological systems (Niesink, Jaspers, Kornet, and van Ree 1999). For most psychoactive substances, an overall career use pattern includes stages of intake, reaction, adaptation, tolerance, maintenance, withdrawal effects, and abstinence. Drugs that cause strong unfavorable reactions after intake may terminate a use career for most users during initiation and experimentation. Drugs that have a long duration of effects may facilitate habituation, and, hence, become prime candidates for career use. Drugs that cultivate adaptation and tolerance may change human biochemical functions and, therefore, perpetuate use through a lengthy career path. For instance, some users shun speed because they are fearful of its uncontrollable effect felt in initial trials. Marijuana smoking develops into habitual career use because marijuana stays long in the body and does not require frequent administration. Smoked crack, with a short duration of rush effects, makes users experience dramatic episodes through career stages, and, hence, drift away from general career pathways. Heroin modifies human biochemical processes in the long run and, therefore, creates physical and psychological conditions for dependent use over the life span. Methadone maintenance treatment provides a medical mirror that reflects the entrenched nature of narcotic addiction.

The general use pattern for each drug can be modified in various forms when applied to individual users in different social backgrounds. Alcohol, coffee, and tobacco are licit substances, widely available in private and public settings. Most people have some experiences with one or all of them in their lifetime. Why do only a certain percentage of people become drinkers or smokers? Among drinkers, why do only a few become alcoholic? Apparently, many individuals are not able to overcome alcohol's "burning" taste or tobacco's "pungent" smell in their initial reactions and, therefore, have only a short-lived career use of the substance. Long-time drinkers or smokers, on the other hand, are likely to have experienced every possible alcohol or nicotine effect—from reaction, adaptation, tolerance, maintenance, and withdrawal, to abstinence—in their use career. With regard to social factors, some long-time drinkers or smokers might have never overcome their initial dislike of alcohol or tobacco on their way to career use if there had not been pressure from their peers, social customs, or culture.

Finally, a particular society or historical era can have a general substance use and abuse pattern in response to its knowledge as well as its legal, social, and cultural practices. Knowledge refers to the inventory of substances known to a society and the level of understanding people have of those substances at a specific time. Legal, social, and cultural practices dictate what substance is controlled and whether a substance is associated with individual status, social functions, life rituals, or cultural ceremonies. The respective histories of alcohol, tobacco, marijuana, opium, coca, and other substances clearly show how people learn about a substance in their natural environment and how they gradually incorporate its use into their social, cultural, and religious activities. Pacific islanders discovered kava from the chewed, pounded, or grated root of *Piper methysticum* on their islands. Over the years, they developed an institution that preserves use of kava as a social privilege to titled or initiated men. Uninitiated, untitled men and members of the opposite sex are either barred from drinking grounds or only allowed to participate in the cultivation of kava plants and the preparation of kava beverages (Lindstrom 1987). Asian mountaineers in the Golden Triangle learned about the opium poppy as it flourishes in their natural environment. Without access to the outside supplies of medicine, they developed a sophisticated system of opium use that serves them to relieve pain caused by hard labor and illnesses (Renard 1996). The New World is a naturally endowed region of hallucinogenic plants. Use of those plants to alter states of consciousness had been important to Amerindian societies long before contact with Europe (Schultes and Hofmann 1979). Among highland Indians, chewing coca leaves entered their Andean culture about a thousand years ago.

In contemporary Western societies, technology, legal regulation, and popular culture converge to complicate the situation of substances, resulting in multiple patterns of use and abuse. Knowledge of natural substances in different parts of the world is publicly available. Imports are facilitated by the advanced means of communication and transportation. Synthetic drugs are manufactured through mass production lines. They proliferate in both open and underground markets. Legally, some substances are controlled. Use of them leads to punishment. Other substances are allowed or protected for use through complicated classification systems. In public attitudes, while many localized groups consider use of some substances as status, maturation, or socially functional, there seems to be a rising suspicion or resistance against any substance use among the populace.

The unique mix of social factors makes it a challenge to identify the general pattern of substance use and abuse in Western societies. First, substances are widely used and abused as they are readily available in natural and synthetic forms, by legal and illegal means, and through domestic and international channels. Second, use and abuse of substances serve multiple purposes, not only for the passive relief from or solution of pain, depression, ambivalence, and problems, but also for the active creation or enhancement of pleasure, euphoria, productivity, and social functioning. Third, use and abuse involve a multitude of substances, from licit to illicit, from mild to hard, and from street to over-the-counter drugs. Fourth, use and abuse of substances figure in all occasions of life, from alcohol at home to coffee during work, from special drugs in private places to beer or wine at social gatherings, and from light dosages on weekdays to a binge over the weekend. Fifth, use and abuse of substances run variably through different age groups. In typical sequences, light drugs and nasal use are mostly associated with youngsters, hard drugs and intravenous use with adolescents, licit or illicit drugs and habitual use with adults, and over-the-counter drugs and dependent use with seniors. Coffee, alcohol, and cigarettes are usually consumed by people of all ages. Sixth, drug use and abuse are marked by differences in social class and status. The poor using cheap drugs in the streets are easy targets or victims of drug overdose and poisoning, police arrests, economic deprivations, crime, and violence. The rich, in contrast, may secure their drug use as a privileged lifestyle through protected sources of supply for a controlled quality of dosage ingredients.

It is obvious that the career perspective sheds light on and provides theoretical images of the general patterns of drug use and abuse among different users, for specific drugs, and in particular societies or historical eras.

Theoretical Components

The career perspective conceptualizes the evolutionary process of substance use and abuse as a career path. It includes three major components in its overall theoretical framework. These components are: career stages, change through career stages, and career roles.

Career Path: Stages of Use

According to the present literature, substance use and abuse progress through initiation, experimentation, casual use, regular use, dependence, and abstinence (Edwards and Lader 1994; Marlatt and VandenBos 1997). The career perspective examines the career path through similar stages. They include nonuse, initiation, experimentation, casual use, habitual use, dependence, and stoppage.

Nonuse. Nonuse is a baseline state, denoting a complete, total, and absolute abstinence from any substance. There are two types of nonuse. One is pristine or virginal nonuse. It refers to never-use over the lifetime. The other is retired or maturation nonuse. It results from past substance uses.

Both types of nonuse are inherently connected to the substance use career. Maturation nonuse is obviously a positive conclusion of a substance use career. Pristine nonuse, while being categorically different from use, supplies possibilities for use. Compared to maturation nonuse, which could be solidified through past use experience, pristine nonuse might be more susceptible to a change into use, especially among young and socially inexperienced people.

Initiation. Initiation is the start of a use career. The circumstance and experience of initiation have direct bearing on the nature of use career. If they are unknowingly brought to a drug scene and develop aversive feelings after first use, users may have a short-lived use and bounce back to nonuse. Initiation can then provide immunity against substance use and lock them into nonuse.

On the other hand, if users are premotivated and have a great deal of interest by themselves, initiation may trigger multiple experiments and lead further to regular use. It needs to be pointed out that veteran users' self-portrayal, media presentation, and political mystification of smoking, drinking, and drug use could fan youngsters' interest in various substances and initiate them into a career of use, misuse, and abuse.

Experimentation. While initiation can be voluntary or involuntary and refers literally only to first use, experimentation is a self-motivated process and may involve a series of use episodes across a considerable time span. The present literature explains experimentation mostly by the physically pleasant experience of initiation (Lowinson, Ruiz, Millman, and Langrod 1992). But many other factors can prompt experimentation as well. For instance, peer influence and social pressure may force people to experiment with some substances even though they gain no pleasant experience from use at initiation.

Through experimentation, users broaden their drug-using horizon, reinforce their positive use experience, develop some coping mechanisms for adverse effects of use, and become physiologically, psychologically, and socially prepared for entry into later stages of career use.

Casual Use. If experimentation takes place sporadically over a wide time interval, users are likely to develop a career of casual use. For alcohol, most people identify themselves as casual, light, or social drinkers. They drink alcohol when they like drinking it, have it at the dinner table, celebrate holidays, or attend social gatherings. In smoking, there are also people who entertain themselves with tobacco occasionally as they please. For marijuana and other controlled drugs, survey data always point to the dominance of casual use over regular use (U.S. Department of Health and Human Services 1993).

What about casual use as a career stage? Does it lead to habitual use? Logically, as casual use gives users all possible experiences of a substance, users may gain immunity against further slide into regular use. However, since casual use does not necessarily rule out occasional problematic use, environmental factors may push users into routine heavy use. For example, some intellectuals report that they initially smoke only when they write and think creatively on research projects. After a concentrated period of work, they automatically become habitual smokers.

Habitual Use. It is possible for habitual use to develop from a period of experimentation or casual use. The apparent indication of habitual use is the regularization of substance consumption in terms of amount and frequency. Using rituals are also incorporated into the daily routine. For instance, drinkers drink at the dinner table, smokers smoke between work intervals, and drug users use controlled substances in a specific time, location, and manner. Most essentially, users' bodily process and rhythm are modified to a degree that regular intake of a substance becomes necessary.

Compared to other stages, habitual use is most stable and lasting. In fact, as other modes of drug-using careers are relatively unstable and likely to develop into regular use, habitual use is often mistakenly equalized to what a whole drug-using career is all about.

Dependency. Dependency begins with habitual use. But as a career stage, dependency signifies loss of self-regulation by substance users over their internal bodily process and external social behavior. As the body loses its elasticity to swing back and forth between consumption and non-consumption, drug users experience more substance craving or obsession than the normal consciousness of human dignity, personal interest, and social responsibility. In fact, when substance craving becomes so overwhelming, they may commit self-destructive or socially violent acts.

In contrast to habitual use, dependence is the watershed where drinkers become alcoholics and substance users turn into drug abusers. As a career stage, it denotes the state of drug abuse and addiction.

Stoppage. Stoppage is nonuse after use. How does use evolve to stoppage? There are several possible routes: death, maturation or maturing out, and quitting. Death is obviously the absolute conclusion of a drug-using career. Maturation builds upon internal changes of drug users over their use career. It may provide a natural exit from substance use. Quitting comes from users' conscious efforts. If those efforts do not endure, relapse can bring users back to their use career.

Stoppage, therefore, can be both transient and permanent. In a full drug-using career, it can be either an absolute conclusion or a transitory state between active uses.

Career Path: Change through Stages

Human beings are material beings. In the sense that life builds upon continuous intakes and recycling of substance and energy, all human beings are realistic as well as potential substance users, misusers, and abusers. It is the result of natural selection and adaptation why some substances are used as foods and medicine while others are identified as poisons, stimulants, depressants, or psychedelic drugs. In concrete terms, using drugs and progressing through use careers are influenced by a host of personal and impersonal factors at physiological, psychological, economic, and social levels (Knipe 1995; Ray and Ksir 1996; Marlatt and VandenBos 1997).

From Nonuse to Initiation. First use of drugs may take place either by accident or as a necessary occurrence. Physiologically, factors contributing to initiation can be genetic inclination, biological-chemical imbalance, food intake, medication, or any other material change that creates a condition of accommodation or craving for the effect of a substance. For instance, people who like the smell of cigarettes or wine are likely to smoke or drink even without any a priori experience.

Psychological factors may include curiosity, excitement, sensation seeking, anxiety, and depression. Curiosity is especially true as psychodrugs are widely mystified by mass media. Teenagers are drawn to their first use often because they are taught to avoid the substance. Customary beliefs also link some substances to a specific psychological state or effect. For instance, people in anxiety may turn to alcohol simply due to the old saying "drink sorrow down" or "drown worry in drink."

Economically, production and trade of alcohol, tobacco, and controlled substances constitute important activities in the market economy. Numerous manifest and latent factors exist to promote initiation to use among youth and habitual use across the population. It is interesting to note that change accumulated by children over a short period of time is often enough to buy their first dose of drug while being seldom enough for a useful possession.

Social factors include influences or pressure from family, peers, school, workplace, and other social network. For instance, use by parents and the availability of a substance at home are likely to initiate an adolescent to use. One social factor that tends to be overlooked is social custom. In primitive societies, youngsters are officially initiated into their adulthood through use of substances, such as alcohol and psychoactive drugs. In industrial societies, the legislation of a legal age has made it a fact that reaching the legal age is equal to initiation into use of alcohol, cigarettes, and other drugs.

From Initiation to Experimentation. This change involves self-efforts on the part of users. Physiological accommodation and adaptations are explored, tested, and developed through repeated experimentation. To most experimenters, motivation for multiple trials comes from the pleasure and changing experience they gain through experimental use. However, there are also cases in which users hope to overcome their unpleasant experience from initial use through continuous experimentation. The key issue is whether experimentation creates a bodily condition of accommodation and craving for a substance. Some physiological characteristics might be facilitative of or amenable to such a condition.

It is also during the changing process from initiation to experimentation that the connection between psychological needs and drug effects is built. Is curiosity served? Does the substance bring about excitement or help alleviate anxiety and pain? Once the connection is established, users may narrow their feelings down to a particular psychological state they expect for themselves. When that state, either aloofness or a sense of attachment, is achieved, experimentation is further reinforced.

Economic factors can be insignificant from initiation to experimentation. First, the cost of use is not high in this period. Second, drugs may be provided free by people under whom experimental users are apprenticed. Third, obtaining a small amount of money for a small dosage from a known or unknown source is relatively easy. Experimentation can sustain well without much risk and cost.

Socially, experimentation can be facilitated by the availability of drugs, the knowledge of drug-using rituals, the network of drug users, and social tolerance or permissiveness. For instance, if drinking or smoking is associated with beauty, celebrity, and a noble lifestyle, new users can be motivated to overcome any resistance to or unpleasant experience from use at physiological and psychological levels through repeated episodes of experimentation.

From Experimentation to Casual Use. Casual use after experimentation is a preferred outcome in contrast to habitual use. If experimentation is intense, casual use may be a proof that users gain an upper hand over the effect of a substance. In physiological terms, they develop tolerance for but have no dependence on it. What physical conditions are necessary? Obviously, a proper level of bodily elasticity is required to accommodate any imbalance caused by the drug effect after use and restore the body to its natural equilibrium when the drug effect is absent in the period of nonuse. By laboratory work, it might be possible to identify and establish the proper level of body elasticity among casual substance users.

Psychologically, change from experimentation to casual use necessitates self-containment of any sensational experience associated with a substance. Users are able to both appreciate the effect of the substance and contain the power of seduction and subjection that comes with their appreciation of the drug effect. Craving is controlled in a way that it is conditioned on the availability rather than the absence of a substance.

Economic conditions can provide underlying motivations for such a psychological adaptation. Saving limited resources and maintaining body sobriety for an income-earning job can strengthen users' free will and lock them into a casual relationship with a substance. Drinking alcohol, tea, or coffee offers an illustration: "I like the effect of high-quality wines, but I can only afford to drink this much of this brand." The same is true for marijuana: "I like the feeling of mellowness after use, but I can live without it for a definite period of time."

Socially, examples of casual use known from the family, neighborhood, school, and workplace can serve users as models for controlled use. Scientific findings about the benefit of light drinking influence people on their drinking behavior significantly as more and more drinkers move toward casual consumption. On the other hand, media mystification of the addictive nature of a substance may create a social conception that simplifies use as dependence and destruction. Once such a general conception is established, casual use seems just impossible as a preferable career use choice. People may, therefore, be socially driven into dependence if they ever use the substance. This is somewhat true for marijuana and other controlled substances.

From Casual Use to Habitual Use. This is a qualitative change. Body elasticity at casual use is permanently replaced with a physiological condition that integrates regular intakes of a substance into the maintenance of the biological-chemical equilibrium. If the mechanism of human evolution provides that sporadic exposures to drug stimulation at casual use trigger bodily adaptations for habitual use, it is then necessary to determine what kind of sporadic stimulations in what frequency could lead to a qualitative change into the regular consumption of a substance.

Psychologically, casual users experience occasional effects in a horizon of noneffect. Habitual users, in contrast, land on a continent of continuous effects dotted only with spots of noneffect. The background changes from noneffect to a constant effect when users seek to amplify the effect of each occasional use or increase the frequency of use at the stage of casual consumption.

In the economic aspect, a direct connection is that increased resources lead to improved access and, therefore, a higher level of use. However, connection can also be built on the opposite. That is, contracted resources knock casual users out of balance, causing irregularity, such as overfeeding after an unusually long period of hunger, in their casual use. A long-lasting irregular experience can then develop into or set a stage for habitual use. Why do affluent middle-class suburbanites drink wine in a casual manner while indigent Indians in reservation camps become drunkards?

Social factors facilitating casual use into habitual use may come from changes in work, study, or interpersonal relationships. Social perception of a substance and its reputation at the level of habitual use can also throw casual users into regular consumption. For instance, smoking becomes a habit for the majority of smokers in a sense that it is so perceived and institutionalized in our culture and society. The same may be true of marijuana as it gains a reputation of being a harmless, beneficial substance amenable for controlled use among the populace.

From Habitual Use to Dependency. Dependency begins at habitual use. It becomes a career stage when use develops into a disease. With dependence, the body is no longer able to incorporate intakes of a substance into its normal functioning. The bodily process is so disturbed that it mistakes handling the substance as its whole function. Timely intakes of the substance, therefore, become a condition to the maintenance of life.

In the user's consciousness, craving for drugs takes the center stage. Desires for physical comfort, personal appreciation, and spiritual elevation are all nullified. The psychological space collapses from its original multiple dimensions into one dimension of consuming drugs and entertaining the effect of drugs.

Dependency can easily drain a user's economic resources. Overwhelmed by constant drug cravings, dependent users are likely to fail in jobs and turn to all possible sources for drug money. Income becomes unstable. Substance intake changes dramatically. Dependency worsens as users struggle repeatedly between overdose and out-of-supply.

In the social aspect, dependence drives users into isolation from work, school, community, and even their family. As they roam in the streets, they are likely to run into trouble with the law. If they are picked up by organized crime groups, they may be used as tools against the mainstream establishment. Substance abuse can, therefore, connect with crime to inflict suffering on both perpetrators and the society as a whole.

Getting to Stoppage. Stoppage can come from any career stage. People use a substance once but never intentionally experiment with it. People experiment with a drug but do not use it thereafter. People use a drug occasionally for some time and stop using it altogether. People maintain habitual use of a substance for a long time and quit their habit forever. People become dependent on a drug and are recovered from it. All of them can gather at the point of stoppage.

At the physiological level, stoppage can take either a voluntary or an involuntary form. Voluntary stoppage does not involve any effort from users. It may occur when some antidrug mechanism is developed after use. For instance, people react negatively to a substance after initiation or experimentation and decide not to use it any more. Stoppage may also occur through a use maturation process by which the effect of a drug becomes gradually nullified, as in the case of casual or habitual use. Involuntary stoppage refers to quitting from habitual use or recovering from dependence through treatment. It takes effect because of medication or other intervention that works to reverse the bodily adaptation to use.

Psychologically, stoppage occurs when users lose interest in the sensational effect brought by a substance. Loss of interest can be caused by long-term exposure, tiredness, and some substitute attractions. However, for stoppage to continue, a new psychological landscape of desires, feelings, sensations, and expectations needs to be in place in the mind of former users.

Economic aspirations may also prevail over the past sensation seeking and solidify the former user's determination with abstinence. Savings from nonuse and earnings from a job can take quitting or recovering users to a new latitude where they see the prospect of establishing economic well-being through hard work.

In the social front, employment is the most important step toward social reintegration for former drug users. Access to social resources and renewal of positive social relations are also important and necessary. To recovering drug addicts who were cast out from the mainstream for a long time, social support can be a determining factor in preserving their newly achieved abstinence.

Career Path: Roles of Use

Different roles of use can be identified throughout a complete career path. It is dialectical that these roles may also reflect particular substance use careers. For instance, casual use can be both a transient role in the developmental pathway of a use career and a lifetime career role. It is, therefore, insightful to examine general characteristics of specific roles in the career path.

Nonusers. Nonusers are people who do not use drugs. There are two groups of nonusers: those who never used drugs and those who used drugs before. In the former, there are drug czars, drug sages, drug idiots, drug phobes, and drug haters who build their abstinence respectively upon power, spiritual sanctity, ignorance, fear, and hatred. Nevertheless, they are all potential candidates for drug use, just like any inexperienced, sensation-seeking, and innocent youngsters who are drug novices but have not developed any particular attitude toward drugs.

In the latter group, there are former drug addicts, casual users, or habitual users. They may either relapse into their past habit or stay clean ever after. Technically, however, retired nonusers may have gained immunity against drugs and can, therefore, be less vulnerable than their never-use counterparts.

Casual Users. Casual users are "take-it-easy" people who probably have the most elasticity in their bodily adaptation. They play normal social roles. They also want to enjoy a few episodes of getaway sensation amid their overall experience of socially approved activities.

Casual users can exhibit a variety of styles in their drug use. They are not just light, occasional, and well-mannered users who condition their drug consumption on a self-regulated routine. There can be occasional heavy users who work in responsible positions on weekdays but indulge themselves in alcohol over the weekend. There can be occasional rule violators who take risks to secure drugs and protect their use in a specific time. Easygoing people who normally do not use drugs may join friends occasionally in a party where they keep smoking, drinking, and using drugs until out of control. To a degree, some casual users can be likened to nasty boys who attend school and do their homework, but nevertheless take enjoyment in being a nuisance in their neighborhood.

Habitual Users. Habitual users are people who integrate regular use of a substance into their bodily process and behavioral routines. The majority are legal substance consumers, such as caffeine users, tobacco smokers, and alcohol drinkers. Habitual users of controlled substances constitute only a minority.

While the majority of legal substance users differentiate by commercial brands, the minority of illicit drug users divide by styles of use. A few privileged persons maintain a style of uninterrupted use as they cherish their deviant idiosyncracy under a supposedly universal curtain of law. These privileged persons may include marijuana users in affluent middle-class communities, hard-drug users among some business tycoons and their profligate children, and controlled substance users among professionals (Coombs 1997). The privileges they have in their life provide them with protective conditions for their drug use career: (a) high income to sustain the costly drug habit; (b) easy access to the higher echelon of dealers in the drug market; (c) a relatively seclusive residence to maintain privacy and protect the drug use lifestyle; and (d) social impressions of celebrity, nobleness, or at least self-sufficiency to avoid attention from law enforcement.

For ordinary illicit drug users who have none of those privileges or protective conditions to sustain their habit, publicly and privately funded maintenance programs in treatment seem to offer a workable, though compromised, alternative. In a sense, delivery of methadone, levo-alpha-acetylmethadol (LAAM), and other medication to poor drug users can be seen as an extension of social welfare in the substance use and abuse arena. Interestingly, maintenance, along with other so-called harm reduction measures, tends to gain more popularity in those European countries where a strong welfare tradition persists (Strang and Stimson 1990).

Problematic Users. Habitual users live with their habit through self-management. However, when physiological, psychological, economic, and social conditions change and run out of control, self-satisfying habits can turn into self-alienating dependence. As dependence takes the center stage, use can become problematic, making users a trouble, a burden, and even a threat to life and property in their surroundings.

Trouble users lose self-control occasionally and charge those who are around them with the management of their problematic drug use. For instance, they may reveal private affairs they share with someone and cause embarrassment; they may become unreasonably provocative and argue with other people; they may throw up and create a mess for the group or family; or they may use their drug habit as an excuse to maintain an abusive relationship with their significant others. Other nuisances they create include: using family grocery money to buy cigarettes, stealing small money to obtain drugs, using family belongings to exchange for drugs, playing on the job, lagging behind schedule, lying on small matters, and so on.

Serious problem users become dependent not only on drugs, but also on family members or other sources for their drug and survival needs. They lose interest in productive social functions and care only about their craving for, comfort with, or suffering from drugs. The level of seriousness in problematic drug use is reflected in two aspects. First, users have no shame in living on public assistance and remain apathetic to how they drain their significant others' financial and emotional resources. Second, users have no sense of bodily well-being and human dignity. They may forget drinking water, eating food, and taking baths. More seriously, they may be unfeeling to various injuries they inflict upon their body through using substances or practicing dangerous activities, such as prostitution and robbery, for drugs.

Violent problem users are epitomized by the violence they commit against people and the damage they inflict upon properties. Driven by their drug craving, violent problem users may join gang groups or drug-dealing networks, and engage in violent crimes, such as robbery, kidnapping, and murder. Under the influence of drugs, they may batter their family members, assault innocent people, and kill themselves and others in automobile accidents. Obviously, violent problem users pose a threat to public safety and a challenge to law enforcement.

Theoretical Applications

The career perspective places the object of study in the time frame of its development to see how it evolves through its natural history, how it relates to its environment over time or at a particular time, and how a particular experience sinks through its whole evolutionary process.

With respect to users, the career perspective requires identifying user statuses over a time span. Are they users or nonusers? If they are nonusers, are they retired or never-use nonusers? If they are users, what type of users are they? Are they novice users, experimenters, casual users, habitual users, or problem users? With status identification, it is then sound to proceed with a biographical analysis of users' drug history. In biographical analysis, users can be studied in detail regarding their initiation, experimentation, use rituals, use routines, and use reactions. Physiological, psychological, economic, and social factors can be related to specific episodes as well as overall development of general use experience. A career profile can, therefore, be established to map the evolution of past drug use and to predict future use or nonuse. For instance, individual profiles on retired users may shed light on whether an irregular exposure to prevention or treatment contributes to withdrawal and what role physiological adaptation plays in the maturation of a drug career. They may also lend some predictability to future use or nonuse behavior.

Regarding a particular substance, the career perspective calls for generalizing from individual user experiences to develop a quasi-career pattern of use or abuse. Is the substance amenable to long-term or short-term career use? Does a general career use involve different stages of progression or regression? What type of users does the substance generate? What kind of overall career path does the substance create for most of its users? With information collected on all these dimensions, a substance profile can be developed. Such a profile may not only serve as a guide for users, policymakers, and concerned professionals, but also provide a basis to study how specific career paths may develop for different users due to their personal characteristics. For instance, while the addictive nature of nicotine promotes a general dependent career use for most smokers, individual career paths still change with user characteristics and differ from one another in terms of style, intensity, duration, and health consequences of use. Legal definitions and the social control status of a substance also matter as social permission tends to steel users toward lifetime use and social inhibition may make a long-term use career unsustainable to most users.

More generally, the career perspective brings about a dialectical approach to time, change, and development involving substance use, misuse, and abuse. Career evolves in time. Time is differentiated by change. Change paves the way for development. Development passes through stages. Concretely, what time frame does a use career involve? Does it correspond to childhood, adolescence, adulthood, or another period of life among users? Does it make a historical era for a substance such as "the heroin era" and "the cocaine era" that have been identified in the United States (Golub and Johnson 1994)? What major stages does a use career pass through? Do all career paths necessarily involve initiation, experimentation, escalation, habituation, dependence, maturation, and abstinence? Or is each use career unique in terms of its evolutionary process? What changes are built into each career stage? Are some changes more important than others? Is there a qualitative change that is primarily responsible for one career stage to develop into another? What are the indispensable agents of change in the development of a use career? Is there any other significant agent of change than those identifiable from physiological, psychological, economic, and social arenas? Is it possible that one agent overrides all others in fashioning an important change in use career development?

Finally, the career perspective creates a possibility to relate substance use and abuse to other career developments in the life of users. With a substance use or abuse career identified, it is natural to ask: What other career series does a user engage in during his or her life? Is there an occupational career, a family career, a career of hobby, a career of criminal involvement, or a career of other interest in his or her life experience? How are these careers related to substance use or abuse unilaterally and multilaterally? Is there a moderation career that regulates substance use or abuse? Is there an acceleration career that fuels substance use or abuse? Or is there a noninteraction career that evolves independently from substance use or abuse?

Empirical Tests

The career perspective creates needs and provides guidelines for empirical research. In designing and conducting specific projects, standard research methods can be employed in terms of their respective applicability, and hence be expanded or enhanced with various new features.

Case studies seem to be most suitable to empirical research on use career. By following individual users through their use career, researchers can develop a user biography, identify major stages of use, and analyze the interplay of use and life events. Similarly, by examining a substance, researchers can establish a use profile, identify a common career path, and analyze how patterns of use change in relation to user characteristics. Methods used in case studies may vary according to research needs. Analysis of archives or documents can be conducted on deceased users. Interviews can be arranged with living individuals. Observation can be used to study behavioral change in or to validate self-reports from a particular case. To establish a substance profile, it may even be necessary to conduct a large-scale survey across the user population as well as some experimental work in the laboratory.

Historical studies fit in well with the time dimension of the career perspective. In microhistorical analysis, historical materials, such as diaries, arrest records, and medical documents, can be used as powerful sources to study the career history for individual users. In macrohistorical analysis, the use career of a substance or a user population is placed in a larger historical context to see how a drug use era emerges from history, how the use career of a substance changes over time, and how a specific user population shape and reshape their use career across different historical periods.

Survey research garners cross-sectional data that can be employed to identify use career patterns in a longitudinal fashion. To study the career use pattern for a substance, it is necessary and efficient to conduct a large-scale survey of current users and to develop a general stage-by-stage pathway for the substance on the basis of user responses. Survey research is also important in supplying information on how a user population are distributed across the main stages of a career span: what percentage of users are initiators, experimenters, casual users, regular users, or dependent users?

Experimental studies can be indispensable and effective to establishing career stages, verifying user statuses, and measuring the effect of an agent on the development of a use career. Scientific experiments in the laboratory can be used to develop a system of biochemical references for different career stages and to ascertain the status of users for accurate diagnoses. In quasi-experimental designs, the effect of a personal or social condition on the progression of a use career from one stage to another can be examined by exposing or withholding that condition to or from selected users at the same career stage and with similar controlled characteristics.

POLICY IMPLICATIONS

The career perspective represents a historical and systematic approach to substance use and abuse. From a historical point of view, it compares substance use and abuse to a career process and studies how use evolves over time. As a systematic approach, it takes substance use and abuse as a whole process and examines how it develops by its own logic as well as in interaction with environmental factors. The career perspective can seriously influence policymakers and practitioners in their decisions on proper reactions and suitable treatments.

Public Health

The primary concern for substance use and abuse from public health is to reduce risk associated with use and render treatment to users as necessary. With a career perspective, health professionals can study common risks associated with a substance and establish a historical curve on how risks or medical conditions change through stages of use. Such a historical curve can provide guidance on when to intervene for risk prevention and where to take action for medical treatment. For instance, risk prevention or reduction may be most effective before or during the stage of use where risk is the highest. Treatment of a medical condition may prove to be ineffective at a stage where it is not yet fully developed. As data on risk and medical conditions for the major substances of use and abuse are collected, health professionals can prioritize their prevention and treatment reactions and focus on those substances that pose the greatest risk and create most medical problems.

With regard to individual users, the career perspective can help health professionals analyze career use pathways, establish use statuses, and identify the prime time of intervention for risk reduction or medical treatment. Previous intervention experiences may also be examined to verify whether timing is important to prevention or treatment. For polydrug users, there might exist multiple use sequences and complicated patterns of interaction among different sequences and substances. However, a historical and systematic analysis can always provide health professionals with a firm foundation for accurate diagnoses and effective treatment planning.

Most important, the career perspective reminds health professionals of the accumulative effect of their intervention efforts on substance use and abuse. Just as use develops through a career pathway, prevention, risk reduction, and treatment build on individual experiences in a historical process. Users may seem inattentive to messages in one prevention, fail on some risk reduction endeavors, or relapse after several episodes of treatment. All these manifestations, however, do not necessarily mean that intervention is useless and users benefit nothing from program activities. In fact, a seemingly unsuccessful intervention may have already helped users pick up some information in their mind and build some latent motivation for change. Through a somewhat stochastic process, a latent effect may manifest itself or may never become manifest. For instance, it may turn up after another intervention, come along with natural maturation, or vanish with death. Health professionals, therefore, should not judge an intervention by its immediate effect nor become disappointed when they see inattention, failure, and relapse following a particular program effort. Similarly, they should not be overjoyed when they see interest, effects, and abstinence after a specific intervention. Instead, they should look at a user's whole experience and see whether effects are differentially attributable to various interventions received across his or her life span. In other words, there ought to be a career perspective to intervention parallel to use and abuse.

Social Control

The present social control reaction to substance use and abuse is universal, lacks specificity, and is overstretched. It is universal because the law that defines an age limit of use and places substances under different degrees of control applies indiscriminately across time and space. It lacks specificity because it does not distinguish among different states of use, types of users, and severities of associated problems. It is overstretched because it reacts to any and all use that is defined as illegal.

With a career perspective, social control can be rationalized, becoming specific, problem-oriented, and effective. First, there should be no universal law on substance and its use. Substance is substance. It can be beneficial or harmful to human beings. If it is harmful, control or legalization can only make its harm more widespread and socially instituted. For instance, definition of a legal age and protected use for adults, as in the legalization of alcohol and tobacco, may inadvertently deprive users of their inner control for dependent use. Likewise, control of marijuana, cocaine, and heroin itself may fuel deviant interest in those substances, unnecessarily creating a menace to the larger society. Without man-made definitions on substance and its use, substance can be what it is by its natural properties. Use can follow its natural career pathway by its own logic. In a socially nonprovocative environment, use may be more casual, self-entertaining, and less problematic.

Second, control should be directed to the consequence of use and limited to problem users. Use progresses through stages and users are distributed across the career pathway. Proactive social reactions may abort use temporarily but may also unnecessarily drag users into problem use. A self-regulated marijuana user, when he or she loses his or her job following an arrest, may develop a problem drug use pattern due to strained income. The problem-oriented control, on the other hand, gives time to use in its natural development and trusts users to resolve problems on their own in their use career. It remains hands-off, though watchful, as long as use does not break out into problems and users stay in line with the law. Problems refer to disruption to social order, violations of the law, commission of a crime, or posing a threat to human life, such as driving under the influence of a substance. The law does not include any status offense about drugs. It is simply about crimes against the person or property, such as stealing valuables for drugs and taking a human life because of drug effects. Within such a legal framework, the career perspective can be especially useful in identifying problem use and users for effective controls.

Third, social control should be synchronized with self-management. Outer containment should be harmonized with inner restraints (Reckless 1961). The human being is a self-adjusting system. Physical discomfort, financial strains, motivation for well-being, and needs for social success can all play out in the long run, making drug users keep their habit in perspective. In fact, problem use represents only an extreme condition and problem users constitute only a minority. Use in most times is self-contained, nonproblem use. The majority users are casual or habitual users who are able to control, manage, and regulate their use hobby or routine through a natural process. On the other hand, inappropriate controls from the outside may not only disrupt inner controls, but also create an adaptive mechanism by which users depend on the external pressure for important self-management processes. For instance, a drinker keeps drinking unless his chattering wife stops him. A drug addict continues using drugs until being taken away by the police or taken care of by social workers as he or she is frequently confronted by them.

Obviously, if social control is not mandated to fight substance use by a man-made law that is based on fear and misunderstanding, it can concentrate on problems associated with abuse. If it targets only problem use and problem users, it can send a message to the majority users that they should use their inner control to manage their use in an orderly and less harmful way. If all users are encouraged to put their inner control, self-management, and self-regulation into full play in their natural use career, social control can then limit its scope, reduce its alienating effect, and develop a dimension of trust, sensitivity, and human touch. With such a perspective, social control can become compact, powerful, and effective in dealing with problems associated with substance abuse in particular and fighting deviance, crime, and destructive behavior in general.

Life and Community

Life is a developing process that involves multiple dimensions of activity. Community provides a communal setting where people interact with one another, creating and maintaining different lifestyles. The career perspective views substance use and abuse as one dimension of life or one element of the community. Use by individuals may come out of choice, needs, or some random effect. The impact on the community may be problematic, unpleasant, and burdensome. But in the long run, substance use and abuse are like any other life events: they just make life and community eventful, dynamic, and rich.

At a more worldly level, the career perspective helps distinguish between transitional and permanent, short-term and long-term effects or statuses of substance use and abuse. With proper distinctions, people can take appropriate approaches toward use and users in their community. First, problem use is temporary. Problem users can come out of the developmental shadow naturally in their use career. The community should, therefore, take a wait-and-see approach, giving users time and letting time heal. While waiting for natural development, members of the community could substitute their moral judgment and negative labeling for care and support to users and their family.

Second, habitual use and some casual use continue on a long-term basis. Some users may manage their use well and pose no danger to people around them. Others may break out occasionally or exist as a continuous nuisance in the community. The key to a proper reaction is, therefore, to view substance use as a lifestyle that, like any other life routines, has the potential to cause problems. Just as a habit of walking a fierce-looking dog in the neighborhood may scare children and leave animal feces all over the place, substance use may cause a secondhand exposure and present a negative influence to children. Members of the community can choose to raise public awareness and fight it as a common problem. They may also tolerate it as a unique lifestyle and compromise their individual preference for overall community harmony.

Work and Organization

Compared to the community that gives refuge to different lifestyles, workplaces are where tasks are performed for productive purposes. Rules should be followed in a way that serves the execution of specific tasks. Substance use and abuse should be dealt with under the same premises. First, is substance use a relevant issue? In some places, use of a substance may be simply irrelevant, such as smoking on a large open farm. If it is relevant, does it impair or enhance job performance? Does it exist as direct or potential hazards to the equipment or workers in the workplace?

The substance profile learned from the career perspective can provide an organization with information to decide whether a substance is relevant in a specific context and whether use should be regulated or not. A substance characterized by a tumultuous use career, if it impairs work performance and poses manifest dangers to the organization, may be prohibited without question. A substance featuring a self-manageable use career, if it does not have any manifest effect on job performance but exists as a nuisance in the workplace, may stimulate a debate on its prohibition. A substance with no detectable side effect from career use, if it enhances productivity or counteracts unfavorable effects from work, may stir a controversy on its promoted use.

With regard to individual users, learning from the career perspective on their use status can assist an organization to make appropriate personnel decisions. If use is prohibited on job, can users be allowed to use off job in the workplace? If use is allowed off job in the workplace, is the organization obligated to accommodate career users with protected areas of use, such as areas for smokers or bars for drinkers? More essentially, how does an organization deal with those employees who are in the heyday of their professional development while passing through the most problematic stage of their substance use career? Should the organization fire them or let them recover from their problem use through sick leave? The career perspective can shed light on those questions by supplying information on whether or not problem use is transitional and moves toward a controllable stage.

It is clear that the career perspective can provide information and justification for regulation or nonregulation of a substance in the workplace. It may also diversify organizational reactions to substance users from intolerance, control, and prohibition to accommodation, noninterference, nondiscrimination, and conditional work relief or on-job leave.

In all, the career perspective examines substance use and abuse as a progression over time. From a career point of view, substance use is not just use of substance. It is distributed across various stages in specific pathways. Substance users are not just users of a common identity. They are differentiated into various roles or statuses through individual careers. Different stages, career paths, and user roles can, therefore, be identified and understood in relation to changes over time and interacting factors across space.

The career perspective has important impacts on the way substance use and abuse are viewed, examined, and handled. With the career perspective, prevention, treatment, law enforcement, and social reaction to substance use and users can become more objective, systematic, and humane. In social intervention, since users at various stages have different needs, an objective need assessment should be conducted to evaluate users in terms of their personal characteristics; their physiological, psychological, economic, and social conditions; and their individual reactions to those conditions. Overreaction from law enforcement may unnecessarily stigmatize novice or self-manageable users and cast them out into dependence or criminality. Similarly, lack of social support for problematic users can unnecessarily increase overall cost from substance-related consequences. It is important to make proper distinctions and direct intervention to where it is needed.

—3—

The Conflict Perspective

Substance use is an individual behavior. However, as it takes place in specific social environments, it connects to larger social structure and process not only in cause, but also by consequence. On the side of cause, conflict within and between individuals and groups; social division between the rich and the poor, the powerful and the powerless, or the educated and the uneducated; as well as tension between human beings and nonhuman existence, may singly or jointly create and maintain conditions for substance use and abuse. On the side of consequence, substance use divides people into contrasting or opposing groups between addiction and abstinence, between dependency and self-sufficiency, between drug users and drug czars, between those who are in need of help and those who offer professional assistance, as well as between the oppressed, the deprived, and the treated and their oppressing, possessing, intervening counterparts. Substance use may also validate, solidify, or accelerate social protest, counterculture, or total retreat from society as a whole.

The conflict perspective views substance, substance use, and substance users as sites, vehicles, or carriers of division, tension, conflict, or confrontation between or among individuals, groups, institutions, social classes, or other identifiable units. They can serve as either means or ends, or become both causal and consequential, both expressive and instrumental, both evaluative and affective in general class struggles as well as specific small-group skirmishes.

SOURCES OF INSPIRATION

The conflict perspective in crime, deviance, and criminal justice challenges the consensus model that members of society by and large agree on what is right and wrong and that law is the codification of those agreed-upon social values. It instead claims that contradiction, conflict, and clash are constant features of human existence and that various interest groups vie to control lawmaking and law enforcement by means of power struggles.

The conflict perspective owes its inspiration to the work of Karl Marx and Friedrich Engels. According to Marx and Engels, the history of all societies is a documentation of class struggles between "freeman and slave, patrician and plebeian, lord and serf, guildmaster and journeyman, in a word, oppressor and oppressed" (1979: 9). Under the capitalist system, the state is organized in a hierarchical fashion to represent not the common interest but the interests of those who own the means of production. Workers, demoralized by capitalist society, are caught up in a process that leads to crime and violence. However, the worst crime of all is the exploitation of workers themselves by the bourgeoisie, the ruling class of capitalism.

Drawing upon Marx's pioneering thoughts, the conflict perspective springs into a wide range of theoretical views and pragmatic positions. The first major group, commonly branded as critical, radical, or Marxist criminology, follows in the footsteps of Marx himself, focusing on the crime-producing nature of capitalist society. Willem Bonger (1916) argued that "the part played by economic conditions in criminality is predominant, even decisive" (669). The capitalist system makes both the proletariat and the bourgeoisie crime-prone, although the former are more likely to become officially recognized criminals. Lower-class individuals come into contact with the law not only because they are deprived of material goods, but also because they are discriminated against by the legal system as targets. Upper-class individuals commit crime when they are pushed by their drive toward success and when they sense an opportunity to make financial gains. Georg Rusche and Otto Kirchheimer (1939) examined forms of punishment in relation to larger social structures. They found that punishments had always been dictated by the modes of production and the availability of labor, rather than by the nature of crimes themselves.

After decades of dormancy in mainstream scholarship, Marxist criminology resurfaced first in 1968, when more than 300 British intellectuals, social critics, and activists attended the National Deviancy Conference to share their disillusion with positivist criminology and to decide on a new direction of study based upon Marxist principles. The conference was followed by a well-constructed publication, *The New Criminology*, in 1973. In the book, Ian Taylor, Paul Walton, and Jock Young declared that class struggles stem from and center around the distribution of resources and power. While the labor forces of the capitalist society are controlled by the criminal law and its enforcement, "the owners of labor will be bound only by a civil law which regulates their competition between each other" (281).

In the United States, a small group of scholars also began to pursue a new radical approach to criminology. At the forefront of the movement were Richard Quinney, Anthony Platt, Herman and Julia Schwendinger, William Chambliss, and Paul Takagi in the School of Criminology at the University of California–Berkeley.

In general, Marxist criminology views crime as a political concept designed to protect the interests of the rich, the privileged, and the powerful at the expense of the poor, the disadvantaged, and the ruled. In capitalist society, despite the existence of apparently diverse interest groups, the only dominant segment is the capitalist ruling class who uses the criminal law to impose its will upon the rest of the population, to protect its material wealth, and to define as criminal any behavior that threatens its favored social order. Specifically, Marxist criminology divides into three camps: instrumental, structural, and dialectical Marxism. Instrumentalists view the criminal justice system as a tool used by the ruling class to control the have-not members of society. As put by Richard Quinney, "criminal law is an instrument the state and the ruling class use to maintain and perpetuate the social and economic order" (1975: 199). Structural Marxism backs away from the instrumentalist position that law is the exclusive domain of the rich. It argues that law and justice serve the long-term interests of the whole capitalist system. As such, the state functions to control anyone, proletarian or capitalist, who threatens its existence (Spitzer 1975). Dialectical Marxism moves further to attend to the effect of the justice system on those who themselves make, enforce, and interpret the law. It points out that the rule of law powerfully conditions the range of possible responses from legal and political authorities.

The second major group is generally referred to as conflict theory. It assumes that deviance and crime result from intergroup conflict and rivalry. Work on culture conflict by Lewis Wirth and Thorsten Sellin represents some of the early contributions in this theoretical tradition. According to Wirth and Sellin, dominant groups impose a vision of cultural reality upon subordinate groups, making the latter and their behaviors deviant, illegal, and subject to punishment. Particular attention was paid to the delinquency of immigrant children caught in a struggle between two cultures (Wirth 1931). Sellin (1938) even extended culture conflict to the process of colonization in which Western imperialists impose their "civilized" outlook upon indigenous cultures in Asia and Africa, subjecting the latter to harsh, punitive control measures.

George Gold (1958) continued the conflict tradition through his group conflict theory of crime and control. He observed that individuals aggregate in groups and groups survive when they serve members well in defending their rights and protecting their interests. For Gold, the entire process of lawmaking, lawbreaking, and law enforcement is a direct reflection of deep-rooted conflicts between interest groups. Every group attempts to marshal support to pass a law in its favor, gain control over the justice system, and curb the interests of opposition groups. Ralf Dahrendorf (1959) proposed a general theory of conflict in human behavior, which later served as a pillar of modern conflict criminology. According to him, people are bound together by enforced constraint, rather than cooperation. Because some people have power and others are subject to it, conflict, disintegration, and change become a constant and consistent theme from society to society.

Inspired by the writings of Gold and Dahrendorf, a number of scholars set out to analyze the role of conflict in contemporary society, specifically how definition of crime favors those who control the justice system. Austin Turk (1969) expanded the conflict approach in the development of his theory of criminalization. He found that, in the application of criminal labels, while dominant groups bound by "social norms of domination" are able to behave congruently with their beliefs, subordinate groups tend to be less sophisticated under "social norms of deference." According to Turk, there are three forms of control: physical coercion, legal images, and living time, and "lawbreaking, then, becomes a measure of the stability of the ruler/ruled relationship" (48). William Chambliss and Robert Seidman (1971) documented how the justice system protects the rich and powerful in their well-respected treatise *Law, Order, and Power*. In America, they asked: "Is the black man who provides such a ready source of cases for the welfare workers, the mental hospitals, and the prisons 'free'? Are the slum dwellers who are arrested night after night for 'loitering,' 'drunkenness,' or being 'suspicious' free?" (503). To them, the answer is obvious: "The freedom protected by the system of law is the freedom of those who can afford it. The law serves their interests, but they are not 'society'; they are one element of society" (503). John Braithwaite (1986) compared differential treatments the U.S. justice system renders to while-collar criminals and petty thieves. The former are least punished despite the fact that their crimes often cost society millions of dollars. The latter receive strict sanctions even though they commit minor crimes out of economic necessity.

The third major group of views and positions within the conflict perspective includes all emerging explanations, from left realism, radical feminism, power-control theory, abortionist and anarchist criminology, and postmodern theory, to peacemaking criminology. Left realism recognizes that the poor and the disenfranchised are not only abused by the capitalist system, but also are victimized persistently by street criminals from their own class (Lea and Young 1984; Schwartz and DeKeseredy 1993). Radical feminism arises along with liberal, Marxist, socialist, and women-of-color feminist theories. It claims that crime against and by women is caused by male aggression, as well as men's attempt to control and subordinate women (Daly and Chesney-Lind 1988). Power-control theory includes gender differences, class position, and the structure of family in the explanation of crime. According to the theory, while lower-class men commit more serious crimes, middle-class youths of both sexes actually have higher overall crime rates than their lower-class counterparts (Hagan 1989). Abortionist criminology shares with anarchist theory in their rejection of state controls. The former advocates a return of power to communities and individuals whereas the latter urges for a formal struggle against the existing system of supremacy through chaos and disorder (Tifft and Sullivan 1980). Postmodern theory focuses on language and communications in legal codes and justice procedures. It notes that those in power can use their own language to define crime and law to the exclusion or dismissal of any opposition group regarding its version of how to think, feel, or act (Arrigo and Bernard 1997). Finally, peacemaking criminology promotes the idea of peace, justice, and equality in society. Viewing the efforts of the state to punish and control as crime-encouraging rather than crime-discouraging, peacemaking criminologists turn to mutual aid, mediation, conflict resolution, and humanist considerations as ultimate solutions to crime and other social problems (Pepinsky and Quinney 1991).

Regarding substance use and abuse, despite its obvious potential to become a powerful framework of explanation, the conflict perspective finds its sporadical applications in only two areas: empirical research and ideological debate. In the former, applications are mostly narrow-minded and specific to particular subjects, variables, or settings, and thus lacking in theoretical depth. There are studies that trace substance use and abuse to localized conflict within the individual, among siblings or partners, or between personal beliefs and social perceptions, between parents and children, and between husband and wife (Rowe and Gulley 1992; Knight, Broome, Cross, and Simpson 1998; Powis, Gossop, Bury, Payne, and Griffiths 2000; Sussman and Dent 2000; Svensson 2000). Research that holds promise to shed light on the influence of social class and other system variables is also generally confined to empirical findings about either particular groups, such as arrestees, prisoners, homeless people, high school students, and professionals, or specific variables, such as family background, income, education, race, and ethnicity (Ringwalt, Greene, and Robertson 1998; Bray and Marsden 1999; Shaw, Hser, Anglin, and Boyle 1999; Sussman and Dent 2000). Not much theoretical generalization is drawn with respect to economic division, cultural clash, racial confrontation, status discrimination, or class struggle in the larger society.

Only in ideological debate, views and positions about drug law, drug enforcement, and drug war seem to lodge in the general dynamics of national or international media, economy, and politics. Some note that control disrupts drug markets. As a result, such markets can be established only by force. Some point out that enforcement disproportionately falls on minorities and immigrants, even though their use of drugs rarely exceeds the norm. Some observe that drug policies and their enforcement lead to political alliances among branches as well as levels of government. In the United States, for example, even though state and local enforcement officials deal with different laws, they all follow their corresponding federal agencies in the level and pattern of enforcement (Meier 1994). Some even draw a parallel between drug war and the holocaust to illustrate how drug warriors approach their prey in the same sequence of actions, from identification, to ostracism, to confiscation, to concentration, to annihilation, as Nazis went after Jews in World War II Europe (Miller 1996). The general theme that fits in well with the conflict perspective is that drug prohibition creates and marginalizes dangerous classes, including minorities, youth, immigrants, and liberals; that drug war generates and spreads antagonism, fear, crime, and violence; and that drug control policies, in the end, serve the whole establishment for political and material gain (Gordon 1994; Meier 1994; Miller 1996).

THEORETICAL FRAMEWORK

The conflict perspective focuses on the conflict aspect of substance use and abuse. Although existing conflict theories lean heavily on social conflict as a cause for deviance and crime, conflict affecting substance use and abuse obviously emerges from sources more than social origin. It also stretches beyond cause, penetrating through process as a parameter of change or crystallizing in consequence as an end state of affairs.

Definition

Conflict refers to the discord of one's feeling or action, the incompatibility of one idea or event to another, the opposition of one interest or principle to another, or the general situation of disequilibrium, disagreement, tension, or confrontation. As far as substance use and abuse are concerned, conflict, no matter whether it serves as cause or consequence, may take a wide range of forms, as contrasting as intrapersonal versus interpersonal, physical versus mental, materialistic versus moralistic, race versus culture, nature versus nurture, group versus class, and community versus society. Within the individual, substance use and abuse may lead to or result from material deficiency, disequilibrium in biochemistry, physical defects, anxiety, stress, or unfulfilled dreams. Between the individual and his or her environment, dispute with parents, siblings, or friends;expulsion from school; layoff by employer; protest against injustice; hostility toward authority; poverty; or imprisonment may lie in the background as a primary cause for or the ultimate consequence from his or her substance use and abuse behavior.

The conflict perspective examines conflict, its escalation and resolution, throughout the whole process of substance use and abuse. In the proper of its theoretical endeavor, it (a) describes and explains various forms of conflict that prompt and intensify substance use and abuse; (b) describes and explains various types of conflict that respond to or emerge from substance use and abuse; (c) identifies and specifies various roles of conflict involved in substance use, control, and treatment; and (d) explores and analyzes how conflict appears, escalates, and persists as well as how it originates, abates, and disappears, pertaining to substance, substance use, and substance users.

Theoretical Image

Substance use is a phenomenon of conflict. Conflict follows and permeates substance, substance use, and substance users at the beginning, throughout the process, and in the end.

Substance is itself a neutral object. But when it comes into contact with human beings, a substance can become a subject of conflict. Old and known substances cling to their established markets, consumers, use rituals, and widespread reputations while new and unknown substances set out to overcome public suspicions, go through testing and questioning, win users, and develop general images. Some substances enjoy protection, status, and glory while other substances receive control, rejection, and demonization. Substances serve to divide and distinguish users as well. Some substances, along with their quality, taste, or appearance, make users look rich, elegant, and powerful. Some substances, through their ingredients, color, or packaging, push users to the rank of the poor, the deviant, and the helpless. For instance, name-brand wine, cigar, and coffee speak more loudly than words about maturity, wealth, power, and privilege just as street-popular glue, speed, and weed do about novice, poverty, deprivation, and disadvantage. Since alcohol, tobacco, and coffee are not only entitled to legal protection, but also deeply rooted in tradition, culture, and social institutions, they are bound to continue or even expand their achieved scale of use, in spite of any exposed harmful effects and expressed social resistance. On the other hand, controlled, evilized, or newly discovered substances, no matter what benefits they may offer to users, are likely to remain in the market periphery, only to the interest of socially marginalized patrons.

Substance use is itself a simple act. But when it takes place in human contexts featuring individual and social perceptions and values, substance use can involve or interact with conflict in all its dimensions. Substance use expresses conflict. The husband sits silently in the corner of the house, with alcohol or tobacco, to vent his unhappiness with his wife. Youths show their disregard for authority through experimentation with drugs.

Substance use results from conflict. People turn to alcohol or drugs when they fail in school or on the job. Teenagers join drug-using peers when they are abandoned by caretakers or run away from home. Substance use leads to conflict. The wife argues with her husband when he throws up from being drunk. Service workers join hands to fight against smoking in bars, restaurants, and other service settings. Substance use intensifies conflict. One falls behind in work and receives a warning from management. As pressure builds up from employment, he or she starts using substances to hopefully enhance his or her performance, to manage a sleeping problem, or to just vent anxiety. Over a period of use, he or she develops symptoms of tolerance, withdrawal, or dependency, or runs into trouble with the law. Following a breakout incident, such as physical collapse and police arrest, he or she loses his or her job. Finally, substance use may also bring conflict into closure. In the simplest scenario, one takes conflict surrounding him or her to heaven when he or she dies from a drug overdose. There are various subtle situations as well. For example, one stops blaming his or her partner when he or she becomes a verified drug dependent. The justice system drops charges against one when he or she enters a drug treatment program for serious drug addiction.

Substance users are not just people who use substances. Among users themselves, they divide by the type, legality, brand, and other properties of the substances they use, by the family, community, or culture with which they are associated, as well as by the education, occupation, income, or status they have attained in their life. Between self-sufficient and trouble-making users of an illicit substance, for example, the former may complain against or express contempt, even hatred, toward the latter for unnecessarily damaging the general image of their favored substance. In the larger society, substance users constitute a general-interest group. They represent specific beliefs, values, interests, fashions, or trends. They compete with or fight against other social forces or groups, periodically or continually, for survival or expansion, protection or influence, and symbolic attention or material resource. In politics, they may advocate for legislation to sanctify use or lobby for public funds to deliver user services. In mass media, they may glamorize substance use by relating it to celebrity, innovation, or liberalism. In trade and consumer markets, they may bargain with every side over every economic issue from access, pricing, quality standard, and licensing, to taxation. In the justice arena, they may refer to addiction and dependency as medical conditions to appeal for treatment in place of prosecution. In public health, they may run into conflict with prevention workers and medical professionals regarding abstinence, moderation, treatment, and recovery. In service and social welfare, substance users obviously compete with many other groups, such as AIDS patients, homeless people, the elderly, or publicly assisted children, for often-limited taxpayer-funded resources.

Across societies, substance, substance use, and substance users high-light, reflect, or signify conflict in various domains and relationships. Be-tween society and its physical environment, substance symbolizes human manipulation of, frustration with, or triumph over nature. While nature offers substances of remedy or solution for various human needs, it sel-dom volunteers a service without strings. A substance having positive use in some areas is likely to cause side effects in other areas. Contradictions consistently feature in human relationships with substances, from foods to medicines to psychoactive drugs. Within society, substance use perme-ates divisions and tensions between ruling and ruled classes, between haves and have-nots, and between conservative and liberal wings. Sub-stance users are frequently denounced as deviants or outcasts, targeted as subjects of coercive control or professional treatment, and blamed for moral decay, poverty, and welfare dependency. Occasionally, they are also glamorized as innovators, criticizers, or conscientious protesters. From society to society, substance use causes friction and confrontation in trade, diplomacy, and political-military maneuvering. Restriction, control, quota, or tariff is imposed, lifted, or relaxed upon import and export of licit sub-stances, including tobacco, alcohol, coffee, tea, and medicines, between nations. Diplomatic protest, economic sanction, military intervention, or political alliance is lodged, staged, or formed in response to transporta-tion of illicit substances, such as marijuana, heroine, cocaine, and synthetic substances, from one country to another. Substance users travel across borders to gain access to drugs on foreign land or to avoid tough restric-tion or harsh penalty for substance use in their home territory. For in-stance, users who develop a substance habit in one society may find it inconvenient, uncomfortable, or even oppressive to live in another soci-ety where substance use is subject to complicated regulation or severe punishment.

Over time, substance, substance use, and substance users receive dif-ferent, often contradictory, treatments from mainstream society. There is a time of noninterference when a substance makes its debut, a group of people use it, and the authority takes no position regarding its use. There is a time of interference when a substance is either medically regulated or legally controlled. Accordingly, substance use is either professionally supervised or arbitrarily prohibited. Substance users are given either mea-sured assistance or outright punishment. Because of the dialectical nature of social evolution, a period of regulation usually leads to a period of deregulation, which then sets the stage for a return to regulation. Between periods of regulation and deregulation, there is a brief time of transition when old forces struggle to maintain their dominance and new forces emerge to establish their influence. Under Western capitalism, for instance, substance use and abuse break out almost epidemically in the stage of capital accumulation when factories are opened up, opportunities are sought after in the frontier, and workers are drawn to industrial establishments or urban centers from rural communities. Widespread use and abuse result in regulation, control, and even prohibition for some substances in a short period of time under some jurisdictions. Substance regulation and control continue and sustain well, despite their arbitrary, coercive, and discriminatory features, during the stage of capital maturation and expansion. Now at the threshold to a new stage of capital appreciation through human growth and technological development, is it possible to overcome contradictions and conflicts so that substances are included or excluded, substance use is adopted or rejected, substance users are respected or warned in the principle of human choice, dignity, and health?

Theoretical Components

The conflict perspective focuses on the contrast of ideologies, interests, and actions among people, groups, agencies, and other social forces in the field of substance use and abuse. In light of conflict, substance, substance use, and substance users are symbols, sites, or bearers of various social contradictions and confrontations, from economic segregation, political marginalization, and cultural clash, to racial-ethnic division.

Substance as Symbol of Conflict

Substance comes from nature. It symbolizes contradictions inherent in the relationship between human beings and their natural environments. Human beings, in their natural adaptation process, continually search for substances for nutritional, medical, decoration, entertainment, and various other uses. While substances offered directly by or made up with materials from nature serve human beings their major purposes, they also bring about various side effects to the human body and mind. Some of them cause bodily ailments. Some of them lead to psychological dependency. In their persistent striving for greater control over nature through science and technology, human beings may be able to better purify a substance, separate it from other substances, change its physical form, alter its chemical structure, contain its effect to a limited area of the body or a targeted function of mind, or even make a new substance using part of an old substance's molecular framework. However, would all these definite human efforts and achievements ever add up to the infinity of nature? The answer is obvious: human beings can know more but can never know all about nature and its various offerings. Predicaments surrounding substances as gifts of alluring benefits or tricks of unavoidable harm by nature will forever accompany human beings as they struggle with nature between dependence and independence, between susceptibility and tolerance, between vulnerability and resistance, between confusion and understanding, and between submission and control.

Reflective of the contradictory relationship between nature and human beings, substance is often used in society to signify problematic situations, such as deficiency, malfunction, lack of control, addiction, and helplessness. Food, beyond its normal intake and function, calls out images of malnutrition, gluttony, or obesity. Medicine is associated with diseases, defects, and disequilibrium. Alcohol implies gratification, indulgence, and evasion of social responsibility. Tobacco is explicitly or implicitly equalized to waste, dependency, and chronic suicide. Marijuana, heroine, cocaine, lysergic acid diethylamide (LSD), amphetamines, and various other illicit substances generate, undoubtedly and immediately, senses or feelings of troublesomeness, self-harm, addiction, deviance, perversion, and hopelessness. To a large degree, substance, when examined critically and contextually, expresses contradiction and conflict between body and mind, needs and demands, expectations and outcomes, means and ends, and eventually individuals and society.

Substance Use as Site of Contradiction

Substance use initiates, reinforces, and follows conflicts between and among various interests, positions, roles, players, agencies, and forces in social life. Typical opposing sides are the young, junior, cared for, treated, supervised, exploited, led, controlled, ruled, or oppressed versus the old, senior, guarding, treating, supervising, exploiting, leading, controlling, ruling, and oppressing camps, groups, or classes.

The socially disadvantaged side voluntarily or involuntarily engages in substance use to gain attention; vent frustration; make a complaint, protest, or rebellion; or retreat from the real world. Young people explore and experiment with new drugs to prove to their old counterparts that they are brave, innovative, and adventurous. Juniors follow substance use rituals and protocols in some professional and recreational subcultures to demonstrate to their senior colleagues that they are mature, know the code of conduct, and are on track to become insiders. Children drink and smoke to deal with the boredom left by their parents' limited involvement in their life. Students use drugs to warn their teachers that they are tired of their teaching and manipulation. Patients overdose themselves to gain attention or relapse from treatment to show to their counselors, therapists, or doctors that they fail on their job duty. Prisoners smoke and use drugs to cope with the reality of incarceration as well as to challenge the control of correctional authority. The unemployed, uneducated, disfranchised, exploited, deprived, or ruled turn to licit and illicit substances as coping mechanisms, expressive devices, or means of protest, rebellion, avoidance, or escape. For instance, high levels of substance use and abuse in reservation camps, inner-city neighborhoods, and ethnic enclaves may mean that people in economically, politically, and culturally disadvantaged positions have lost their basic hope in the general social system.

The socially privileged side, on the other hand, intentionally or unintentionally deploys or employs substance use to gain status, divert public attention, justify control, create panic, or advance their own position. In participating in substance use, the old, the rich, the informed, and the powerful show their experience, wealth, knowledge and skill, authority, and status with high-quality name brands of substances that are preciously made, delicately packed, imported or gathered from exotic or dangerous sources, and off limit to the populace. Even in the use of commonly known substances, seniors tend to create awe in juniors by telling tough stories, offering technical tips, or implementing rites of passage. Most revealing and dramatic, however, is the fact that the dominating side demonizes, denounces, rejects, and fights substance use while using it as an excuse or reason for control and punishment. Parents tell children that substance use is bad. They ground, shame, or abandon their children when they smoke cigarettes, drink alcohol, or take illicit drugs. Teachers teach students that drug use is illegal. They lecture, suspend, or expel their students when they are caught in drug use. Counselors, therapists, and doctors approach substance use as a problem, disorder, disease, or chemical dependency. They need and use substance abuse clients or patients as their experimental sites for new methods of treatment and therapy. Conservatives argue that substance use is immoral. They agitate for abstinence and drug war in the media and through the community network. Politicians condemn drug abuse as a social problem. They campaign for tough legislation and swift justice reaction in state capitals, city halls, public rallies, as well as on diplomatic missions. Justice officials look for drug use and violations from place to place. They question, search, arrest, and punish people involved in drug use, possession, and transport on a daily basis. Given all these diverse forces and orientations surrounding substance use, it is possible that substance use is created or blown out of proportion as a social menace even though it is in fact not a serious problem. It is possible that substance use is used by some interest groups to shirk responsibility, avoid real issues, and manipulate public opinion. It is possible that substance use is deployed by media, economic, and political stakeholders to quiet critics, control troublesome populations, and maintain the status quo as the favored social order. It is no surprise, from a conflict point of view, that one group finds themselves first drugged, then demonized and punished, and eventually deprived, disfranchised, or disengaged from the mainstream society by the government or by an opposing but dominating group.

Substance User as Creator, Messenger, or Victim of Confrontation

Substance users are both active and passive agents in the use of substances or in the process of substance use. On the active side, they use substances. They are subjects of substance use. On the passive side, they suffer from the addictive power and other harmful effects of substances. They face moral, legal, and social consequences from substance use. If it is said that substance is a symbol of conflict and substance use is a site of contradiction, it is only natural to assume that substance users are creators, messengers, and victims of confrontation.

As creators of confrontation, substance users engage in substance use to produce, verify, solidify, or escalate conflict situations. Within themselves, they drink to create a hangover. They smoke and use addictive drugs to produce a withdrawal syndrome. While they may manage anger, frustration, or stress as fleeting mental states, they become drunk and drugged to make those transient feelings verified and solidified problems. Various originally manageable nuances develop into full-blown conflicts when users turn to substances for temporary relief or escape. Beyond themselves, substance users consume tobacco products to cause long-term secondhand smoking effects for their spouses. They binge on alcohol, prompting their parents to change their attitude from unexpressed dissatisfaction to open distrust and loss of hope. They use illicit drugs to turn themselves from low academic performers to school dropouts. To the larger society, substance users, by the medical conditions they have, the safety hazards they present, the moral danger they epitomize, and the social disruptions they pose, make themselves a challenge to face, a target to attack, an enemy to fight, and a problem to be dealt with by medical professionals, justice officials, conservatives, and politicians.

As messengers, substance users explicitly and implicitly speak about fundamental contradictions and divisions in human life and across societies. Explicitly, substance users tell stories through the mass media and academic studies about the pain and suffering they experience within themselves, as well as with various forces in their environment, prior to, during, and after substance use. Implicitly, substance users signify underlying conflicts and problems in the human body, human mind, social relations, and natural-cultural-political-economic environments. For instance, some people are more inclined to use and abuse certain substances because they are born with specific genetic defects or grow up with particular mental conditions. Some people tend to habitually or problematically consume certain substances because they live in some climates or reside in some parts of the world. Some are more susceptible to substance use and abuse because they suffer from abusive relationships with parents, spouses, or friends. Similarly, a high level of substance use and abuse among newcomers, minorities, the poor, the uneducated, the unemployed, the controlled, and welfare recipients speaks more pointedly about cultural hostility, racial division, economic deprivation, political alienation, and social discrimination in the larger system than anything else.

As victims in social confrontation, substance users become scapegoats for financial stress, budget shortfall, business slump, political corruption, professional incompetency, cultural poverty, moral decay, urban decline, and various other problems at local, regional, national, and international levels. Some typical blames fabricated and forced upon substance users include: they drain government budgets; they overload the justice system; they overwhelm medical facilities and social service agencies; they allure and bribe politicians and justice officials; they scare away customers and business owners; they are responsible for downfalls in morality, culture, and a whole neighborhood, city, or society. From a critical point of view, however, all these blames can be met with logically sound and solid counterarguments. For example, substance users are used by the government to increase spending on equipment, office amenities, salary, and personnel. They are used by the justice system to cover up its inadequate response to crime: instead of sharpening their skills to catch and prosecute real criminals, justice officials keep arresting and harassing substance users to meet their performance quotas. They are used by medical and service staff to mask their professional incompetency: instead of searching for effective treatment methods, medical and service personnel condescend to substance users as incorrigible, incurable, and helpless addicts and junkies. Most critically, substance users may be wrongfully charged by politicians, business owners, church leaders, cultural critics, and local residents for whatever loss, failure, and problem they are not able to deal with in their own capacities.

Conflict Typology, Nature, Initiation, Escalation, and Resolution in Substance Use and Abuse

Conflicts involving substance, substance use, and substance users vary in type and nature. There are intrapersonal conflicts between body and mind, as well as among different areas, parts, and functions of the human body or mind. There are interpersonal conflicts between parents and children, teachers and students, supervisors and workers, as well as among relatives, friends, neighbors, peers, and co-workers. There are intra-agency conflicts, between prevention and intervention, detection and investigation, prosecution and adjudication, rehabilitation and punishment, counseling and self-help, as so often exposed in the criminal justice system. There are interagency conflicts between work and community organizations, justice and medical establishments, and research and policymaking entities, as well as among various governmental and service agencies. The nature of conflict can be personal, direct, emotional, and intense, such as conflicts between parents and children and between counselors and clients. It can also be indirect, institutional, general, and even conceptual, such as conflicts between the mainstream culture and drug subcultures, conservatives and liberals, and politicians and antiestablishment elements, as well as among substance user groups, law enforcement agencies, and service professionals.

Despite its diverse types and features, conflict surrounding substance use and abuse follows two general routes in initiation, escalation, and resolution. On the one hand, conflict makes its onset when substance use is initiated. It escalates as substance use intensifies. It abates when substance is controlled, substance use is regulated, and substance users are circulated out of the population through treatment or institutionalization. It comes to a closure when substance users pass away or revert to abstinence. On the other hand, substance use takes place when conflict breaks out. It increases when conflict worsens. It decreases when conflict dissipates and lessens. It would disappear should conflict ever be eliminated from human life. The two general routes of change between conflict and substance use obviously manifest in various concrete forms under specific situations involving particular substances and users. To the extent that conflict goes hand in hand with substance use as each other's cause, reinforcement, and consequence, the relationship between them is itself a contradiction inherent in human existence.

Theoretical Applications

Approaching substance use as both subject and object of conflict, the conflict perspective opens up a number of questions for theoretical exploration.

Beginning with substance use as the subject of conflict, why are some substances more likely than others to cause addictions, controversies, and problems? Are there any unique factors in chemical composition, pharmacological properties, marketing practice, control status, or public perception that explain why one substance is more prone than another to fall under conflict situations? Use itself may also be critically scrutinized in terms of time, location, and other essential features. For instance, is substance use more likely to be targeted for criticism, condemnation, shaming, or control when it takes place on weekdays than on weekends, during work than on vacation, at collective gatherings than in solace, in freedom than under incarceration, with prescription than without prescription, and under supervision by medical professionals than with drug-using peers? Similarly, substance users may become differentiated in conflict by age, race, gender, and various social characteristics. Are young, minority, female, poor, abandoned, unemployed, homeless, and disadvantaged substance users more likely to be stigmatized, punished, or distanced than their old, majority, male, rich, protected, employed, sheltered, and privileged counterparts?

Regarding substance use as the object of conflict, can conflict be legitimately distinguished among the substance-prone, neutral, or substance-inhibitory? In a substance-prone conflict, are substances brought to the scene of conflict widely available or legally controlled? Are some substances more likely than others to be featured in conflict and stress? For instance, alcohol is used in interpersonal argument. Marijuana is used in terminal diseases with enormous pain. Coffee is used in increasing amounts when workload looms large before a deadline. With respect to use, is substance abuse impulsive, situational, habitualized, or ritualized? Does substance use exacerbate, lessen, or have no bearing on the existing conflict? For instance, a man drinks alcohol whenever he argues with his wife. In the beginning, alcohol use seems to reinforce his anger and tension with his wife. However, since it has gradually become his routine or ritualized reaction to spousal conflict, alcohol use actually helps him cool off from further confrontation. Finally, are substance users active agents seeking substances as ways and means to avoid, alleviate, or manipulate conflict? Or are they just passive recipients when substances are forced upon them? For instance, is it true that veterans suffering from certain battlefield syndromes are administered some allegedly safe and useful medications so that they can remain trouble-free from the government? How much credibility is there in the seemingly improbable conspiracy theory that the minority, the powerless, or the have-nots are induced into drug use, abuse, and addiction by the majority, the powerful, or the haves so that they can be legitimately controlled or treated from making any disruption to the social order?

Empirical Tests

The critical perspective requires a critical attitude toward various social roles, agencies, forces, and their interrelations involved in substance use. Only with such an attitude can significant issues and ideas be identified for serious scientific scrutiny.

Case studies are suitable to tracing intra- and interpersonal conflict and its interaction with substance, substance use, and substance users. At the center is the chicken-egg question: does conflict cause substance use or does substance use lead to conflict? Focusing on a particular substance, case studies can verify whether the substance is generally used only when biological defects, mental disorders, or interpersonal conflicts are present. Following various specific types of substance use, case studies may explain why binge, use at the party, unsupervised use, intravenous use, use in combination with other drugs, or irregular use is more likely than piecemeal use, use with personal discretion, supervised use, nonintravenous use, use without drug interaction, or habitual use to cause problems. Most important, individual users can be studied to detail if one uses substances due to a physical ailment, a mental condition, or constant conflicts in life or at work; how conflict develops in his or her substance use career; and whether he or she is able to manage or manipulate conflict in the process of substance use.

Historical analysis is appropriate when a historical era or a large social system is involved. Documents and statistics can be gathered to demonstrate a long-term developmental trend or prevailing system pattern regarding conflict and substance use. Is substance a center of interest or a collateral issue in trade war, military intervention, diplomatic friction, or hostage crisis? Does substance use serve as a means of discrimination, subordination, and control by the rich, powerful, and educated against the poor, powerless, and uneducated? Are substance users active agents in social change? Or are they just passive recipients of all possible treatments from society: sympathy, care, and rehabilitation on the one hand, and denouncement, avoidance, and abandonment on the other? For instance, a valid historical analysis can be conducted to show how drug war draws negative attention to historically and institutionally disadvantaged groups while channeling resources to politically, culturally, and professionally protected sectors, such as law enforcement, mass media, social service, and medicine.

Survey research is essential to gathering attitudinal and behavioral information from different social groups about substance use and abuse. Are there misperception, misunderstanding, and mistreatment among politicians, justice officials, service personnel, or medical professionals toward substance use and substance users? Are there significant differences across age, gender, education, occupation, income, race, and ethnicity in personal dissatisfaction, interpersonal conflict, social stress, and substance use? Specifically to substance users, do they experience more conflict than nonusers? Are they conflict dodgers, manipulators, or managers as substance users? How do they perceive life, work, society, and the world? Is there an excessive level of distrust, suspicion, and hostility among substance users in dealings with people and institutions in their social environment? By asking proper subjects appropriate questions in large-scale surveys or face-to-face interviews, substance, substance use, and substance users can be studied in all possible associations with disorder, stress, conflict, and problematic situations.

Experiment is needed to determine the causal relationship between physical defects or mental disorder and substance use. Taking defects or disorder as instances of conflict or stress, researchers can use laboratory tests to measure the severity of a particular condition, ascertain the aftermath situation of a specific substance intake, and establish possible links among physiological, psychological, and pharmacological variables. In quasi-experimental designs, parental separation, foster-home care, lack of education, joblessness, homelessness, neighborhood violence, peer pressure, and poverty can be related to substance use in varying situations to see if the former causes or reinforces the latter, or vice versa. For instance, children of divorced or incarcerated parents can be compared to children living with both parents to verify whether parental absence as a situation of conflict or stress is more likely to result in substance use and abuse. Since parental absence is where a child's conflict with his or her parents becomes absent or is replaced by some other contradictions, it may also be interestingly studied as an instance of nonparental conflict or parental conflict substitution. At any rate, experimental and quasi-experimental designs afford researchers various comparative conditions to examine conflict and substance use as each other's cause or effect.

It is obvious that analysis and argument using the conflict perspective can go beyond ideological overtures as so often associated with the perspective under conventional wisdom. They can firmly lodge in rigorous scientific research featuring methodically valid and reliable design, experimentation, data collection, data processing, modeling, theorizing, and interpretation.

POLICY IMPLICATIONS

The conflict perspective views substance use with a critical lens. It takes critical courage to attend to and act out of practical suggestions derived from the perspective.

Public Health

While health professionals are trained to diagnose and treat physical defects and mental disorders with substances, they are not necessarily socialized to view and interact with their substance use clients in any critically thoughtful manner. Most of them are not always aware of the conflicting interests of the different parties involved in their practice. They probably do not spend much time contemplating how conflicting forces in their professional dealings figure in to affect the quality, mode, and delivery of care, service, and treatment they provide for their patients or clients.

With the conflict perspective, health professionals can look at their substance use clients and patients in relation to different people and social forces in the larger system. By recognizing the conflict their clients and patients have with family, school, employer, media, welfare, and criminal justice, they may be able to assume a morally reasonable, emotionally sensitive, and socially responsible position toward substance use and users. For instance, they can join other social forces in advocating treatment instead of punishment for illicit drug abusers. By understanding various conflicts their clients and patients have to deal with in life, health professionals can find sources of inspiration for innovative and effective methods and procedures in diagnosis, prevention, and intervention. Treatment programs, such as group sessions, therapeutic community, family counseling, and vocational training, are developed in response to specific problems. They can only be improved and redeveloped by studying the often conflicting experiences of clients and patients.

Most critically, health professionals need to recognize and admit the conflict they themselves have with their clients and patients. At the outset, they normally view their clients and patients as objects, targets, and challenges to treat, conquer, and deal with. They identify health conditions, creating and issuing labels, such as disorder, addiction, and relapse, for those who happen to have a health condition. They prescribe medications, dictating who obtains what substance in what frequency for how long. They design treatment, imposing not only behavioral but also attitudinal restraints on clients and patients. There are abuse, mistreatment, and malpractice. But when unfortunate events happen, medical boards and other health establishments are likely to side with health professionals at the expense of clients and patients. To patient families, the government, media, and funding agencies, health professionals tend to intentionally and unintentionally present the most severe situation or the worst scenario of their substance use clients and patients. By doing so, they gain attention, respect, and resources for their practice, while unnecessarily tarnishing the general reputation of their clients and patients, and their substance use lifestyles.

What does the conflict between patient-clients and health professionals mean to health care and service? Since health professionals are on the side of power and control, should they be subjected to higher moral standards and more stringent codes of conduct in professional practice? If they should, who would act as a relatively neutral party to broker an assumed fair relationship between patient-clients and care-service providers?

Social Control

The relationship between social control agents and substance users is known to be adversarial. In the eyes of social control agents, substance use is a questionable, potentially dangerous, or outright rule-breaking behavior. It is to be regulated, monitored, or controlled. Substance users are troublemakers, deviants, or law violators. They are to be watched, supervised, or caught. Social control agents are naturally poised to use tricks, forces, and other control measures to deal with substance use and users.

At the outset, the conflict perspective can reinforce social control agents in their vigilance against substance use and users because it warns them how substance use may run wild in disrupting social order and how substance users may attempt everything possible to run away from their detection, investigation, and intervention. With a reinforced vigilant mentality, social control agents may go further to develop deeper suspicion toward substance users and adopt more dramatic strategies in fighting substance use. The outcome is then obvious: more frequent and intensive conflicts between social control agents and substance users.

Instead of leading to greater social division, the conflict perspective may also result in better social cohesion. First, given the fundamental conflict social control agents have with substance users, some due process procedures may be instituted to protect substance users in their basic human rights and civil liberties. Police brutality, judicial biases, correctional abuse, and bureaucratic repression can be routinely reviewed and handled by some impartial groups composed of experts, civilians, professionals, social control agents, and civil rights advocates. Second, social control agents may come to understand why substance users hold hostile attitudes toward and even take dangerous actions against them, when they know what needs and interests substance users have and how substance users are forced into the corner through cultural stereotyping, political repression, economic deprivation, and social discrimination. Third, social control agents may look into the conflicts substance users experience with various parties in their environment. By resolving one or two of those conflicts, they may automatically save themselves from attacking substance users as their ultimate targets.

Life and Community

The community provides a refuge where substance users, along with their neighbors of various lifestyles, express their feelings, meet their needs, and pursue their interests. Recognizing the generally hostile and often repressive measures taken by the outside social agencies, such as drug control and treatment authorities, toward substance users, the community may conspire to act as a safe haven of protection, a source of understanding, or a buffering zone for substance use and those who practice it. The exact reaction of a community depends upon the nature of the community itself. If the community as a whole has been a target of criticism, discrimination, or racial profiling by mass media, social welfare, or criminal justice, it is likely to align with its individual members to fight their particular arrests or punishments as a common threat.

While it may act as a united entity to the outside, the community divides into different interests and camps within itself. There are people who advocate substance use. They view substance use as their neighbors' personal right and lifestyle choice. They emphasize the benefits of substances to human mind and behavior. There are people who sympathize with substance users. They look into various personal circumstances experienced by substance users. They attempt to understand why their neighbors are lured, prompted, or forced into substance use by hope, temptation, failure, suffering, or relational trouble. There are people who oppose substance use and hate substance users. They describe how substance use attracts drug dealing and gang activities, ruining public safety and security in their neighborhood. They detail how substance users party late and loud, cause traffic accidents, create secondhand exposures, and produce many other nuances upsetting them as neighbors from time to time. Substance use hence remains an issue of concern, debate, or confrontation within the community as groups and forces involved vie for recognition, support, and dominance.

It ought to be pointed out that a community can be easily coopted by the authority when antisubstance sentiments prevail and use is generally perceived as a deed of evil by the majority of the community. In cooption by the authority, the community may not only open itself up for external intervention, but also volunteer information leading to the investigation, arrest, or prosecution of some of its allegedly wayward members.

Work and Organization

The interests of an employment organization are to hire and keep qualified employees who perform their assigned duties with competence. When an employee is found to have substance use problems, the employer may either "cover it up" or "cut it off" to avoid negative publicity and possible disruption to business. In "cover it up," the employer may work with the employee to downplay the problem in front of the public, protect evidence from the police, seek professional assistance, and fight prosecution through every legal avenue. In "cut it off," the employer may use the employee's problem with the substance or fiasco with the law to sever its relationship with him or her. The message sent by termination can be clear and loud: the employee is solely responsible for his or her substance use problem and the company has nothing to do with it, not a single part of it.

In recent years, more and more work organizations have responded to the government in its calls for drug testing, employer assistance, and other on-job substance service programs. Why did most employers not resist the government in implementing those programs? They could well fight it, accusing the government of unnecessarily shifting moral responsibility to civilian organizations. The answer to the question, as well as to the questions of whether those programs continue and for how long, lies in how various employment organizations perceive their fundamental interests and how they relate their own needs to general social responsibilities. For instance, as long as substance use is portrayed as a society-wide challenge, many employers will be willing to conduct drug testing to screen out drug-abusing employees who could someday fail on job, bring damage to company reputation, or drain organizational resources with their personal problems. Employers will also be willing to offer various forms of employer assistance, such as sick leave, on-job counseling, or paid treatment, if they find each of them cost-effective in retaining an experienced, loyal, and productive employee team. On the matter of licit substance and its social use, some employers may provide morning coffee, deliver specific job-hazard-resistant substances, designate smoking areas, or organize employee get-togethers featuring alcohol use when they see some of those measures help soften organizational image, improve employee relations, or promote employee identification with the company.

The conflict perspective obviously sheds light on how a work organization perceives and pursues its interests regarding substance use and abuse in agreement or conflict with various other interests, such as those by the board, the government, the union, and the community.

Generally, substance, substance use, and substance users can be examined as sources, centers, or consequences of conflict. From a conflict perspective, substance signifies not only the contradiction inherent in human adaptations to the environment, but also the conflict between body and mind, between nature and nurture, between need and enjoyment, between performance and entertainment, and between various other contrasts in life. Substance use may originate from physical defects, mental disorders, personal stress, or problems in the family, school, employment organization, community, culture, or general social system. It may also exist as a cause of concern, trouble, disruption, or turbulence in personal, racial, institutional, cultural, and other domains. Substance users, out of their engagement in or commitment to substance use, may represent particular voices, ideologies, values, interests, or forces in social dynamics. Posing a challenge to long- or widely held beliefs and norms, they are natural targets for traditional, conservative, or mainstream criticism and condemnation. Existing as a possible threat, disruption, or danger to social order, they become easy prey for criminal justice officials, medical professionals, and service personnel in their efforts of punishment, treatment, and rehabilitation.

The conflict perspective identifies and analyzes essential needs and interests of various social roles and forces involved in substance and substance use. It shows how conflict and substance use are embedded in interests, how they relate to each other through interests, and how they each originate, escalate, abate, or disappear when people, social institutions, and their interests change from time to time.

— 4 —

The Functionalist Perspective

Substance use and abuse take place from group to group, society to society, and generation to generation. No matter whether they are allowed or prohibited in particular societies or historical periods, substance use and abuse are always part of social life, cultural practice, and general human survival in and evolutionary adaptation to the environment.

The functionalist perspective examines substance use and abuse in the context of the larger social system. In general, it explores how substance use and abuse are necessitated by a social system and what they offer to the functional operation, maintenance, and progression of the social system, once they occur and exist, either in the form of deviance or under the appearance of normality. Specifically, the functionalist perspective studies substance intake, substance users, and substance use in respective relation to the human body, individual groupings, and the sociocultural system. It attempts to offer critical insights into how the former contributes to the latter in various functional aspects.

SOURCES OF INSPIRATION

The sociological tradition of functionalism began with Auguste Comte (1896) when he envisioned sociology as "the investigation of the laws of action and reaction of the different parts of the social system." Herbert Spencer (1896) put forth the concept of differentiation in his evolutionary theory. By differentiation, he illustrated the important aspect of a social system's interrelatedness and integration. Vilfredo Pareto patterned society on a physiochemical system characterized by interdependence of parts and adjustive changes (Finer 1966). He was the first sociologist to provide a precise description of how a social system adapts and changes while maintaining equilibrium.

Despite early insights, functionalism emerges as a leading theoretical paradigm in contemporary sociology mainly through three sociologists and their respective contributions. First is Emile Durkheim and his pioneer studies of anomie, suicide, religion, and social integration. Second is Talcott Parsons and his grand theory-building concerning system levels, individual actions, pattern variables, functional system problems, and social change. Third is Robert Merton and his clarifications of dysfunction, manifest and latent functions, and functional alternatives. As a whole theoretical perspective, functionalism emphasizes and is interested in studying: (a) functional interdependence of parts to maintain social structure; (b) group norms to maintain social order and stability; (c) societal equilibrium built upon consensus, conformity, and adjustment among social constituents; and (d) deviance and social pathology resultant from maladjustment of social units (Wallace and Wolf 1995).

Regarding deviance and social pathology, Durkheim (1964) considered them normal because they are universal, present in all or the majority of all societies, and necessary, needed for the continued existence of society. For example, crime is normal because "crime is present not only in the majority of societies of one particular species but in all societies of all types" and because crime is "an inevitable, although regrettable phenomenon, due to the incorrigible wickedness of men . . . a factor in public health, an integral part of all healthy societies" (Durkheim 1964: 67). Specifically, Durkheim pointed out that deviance contributes to social order in several ways: by setting moral boundaries, strengthening in-group solidarity, allowing for adaptive innovation, and reducing internal societal tensions.

Parsons viewed deviance as both generating its own control and renewing a system's equilibrium. According to him, people conform to law and order because they are taught to do so through three mechanisms of social control: socialization, profit, and persuasion. Deviance occurs when socialization is imperfect, profit is lacking, and/or persuasion is weak. There are two types of deviance. Active deviance involves a direct rejection of conformity, resulting in hostility and aggressive behavior toward society, as demonstrated by the actions of protesters and revolutionaries. Passive deviance involves an indirect avoidance of responsibility, leading to withdrawal from a productive lifestyle into a world of madness, as illustrated by the life of alcoholics and drug abusers. To curtail the force of disorder caused by deviance, the state and other forms of authority may apply coercion as a necessary and legitimate mechanism of control to restore social equilibrium (Parsons 1951).

Merton (1957) studied the corrupt big-city political machine. He noticed that deviance can be functional to some units while dysfunctional to others because not all social units are harmoniously integrated in the system. To any specific unit, deviance can be both positive and negative. It is therefore critical to examine the "net balance" of a deviant act's functional contributions. Also, not all functions are recognized and intended. Researchers should be cognizant of various unrecognized and unintended functions by deviance. Most important, Merton provided five general guidelines for the study of deviance: (a) describe the specific form of deviance being studied; (b) identify the range and type of alternatives excluded by the dominant pattern of deviance; (c) assess the meaning of the deviant activity for those involved; (d) discern the motives for conforming to or deviating from a particular dominant interaction pattern; and (e) describe patterns not recognized by participants but that appear to have consequences for the particular individuals involved and/or other patterns or regularities in the wider social context (Merton 1957).

Following Durkheim, Parsons, and Merton, a number of studies attempt to identify specific types of deviance and pinpoint their respective contributions to social order. Robert Dentler and Kai Erikson (1959) studied deviance in groups. Applying a variety of fieldwork techniques to the study of Quakers as well as trainees in the U.S. Army, they gathered data illustrating positive consequences of deviance for the organization. Between the two groups they studied, they found (a) groups tend to induce, sustain, and permit deviant behavior; (b) groups tend not to alienate a member whose behavior is deviant; and (c) deviant behavior functions in maintaining group equilibrium. Continuing his research into the function of deviance, Kai Erikson published his work on the Puritans of the Massachusetts Bay Colony in 1966. First, he observed that "each time the community moves to censure some act of deviation, it sharpens the authority of the violated norm and restates where the boundaries of the group are located" (Erikson 1966: 13). Second, he noticed that "it is not surprising that deviant behavior should appear in a community at exactly those points where it is most feared. Men who fear witches soon find themselves surrounded by them; men who become jealous of private property soon encounter eager thieves" (Erikson 1966: 22). Finally, Erikson (1966) found that society channels certain of its members into relatively fixed careers in deviance to generate something like "quotas" of functionally needed deviants.

Kingsley Davis (1971) studied prostitution. Under the assumption that there is a higher male need for sexual adventure, he argued that prostitutes help men channel their excessive male sexual drives without getting them connected with love. A division of affection, which would inevitably occur when a man is pushed by his greater sexual needs toward another "eligible" woman outside the marriage dyad, is prevented as he meets his sexual needs instead through a "noneligible" female, the prostitute, who exchanges sex not for love but for money. Emotional bonds between husband and wife can therefore be preserved, which in turn will lead to lower rates of marital conflict, divorce, and societal instability. In a similar line but without Davis's obviously sexist assumption about unequal sexual drives between men and women, a few researchers examined swinging or mate swapping to the contention that it sustains the sentimental bond of marriage by providing participants an opportunity to release their marriage-threatening sexual fantasies for an evening or weekend (Denfield and Gordon 1970; Walshak 1971).

Regarding substance use in particular, an early, commonsensical, and consistent note of function is on recreation or pleasurable effect. People use substance to escape from hardship, to relieve boredom, or to gain attractive experience (League of Nations 1930; Lowinson, Ruiz, Millman, and Langrod 1992). Psychologists are the first groups of scholars to view alcoholism and drug addiction as responses to depression, strain, tension, or anxiety. Through psychological work, it is generally recognized that drinking, drug assumption, and other addictive behavior serve to address fundamental psychological needs (Maurer and Vogel 1954). Anthropologists attempt to examine substance use in relation to economic survivals, cultural practices, and environmental adaptations. Sociologists join in the effort by focusing on systemic variables such as anomie and social integration. Donald Horton (1943) cataloged the functions of alcohol in primitive societies, suggesting that the strength of the drinking response in any society tends to vary directly with the level of anxiety in that society. Charles Snyder (1964) used rates of alcoholism as an indicator of anomie and made a bold inference about a lack of anomie among Jews, whose rate of alcoholism is negligible. Judith Adler (1966) urged a full inspection of functional equivalents to alcohol and drug assumption, such as gambling and sexual perversion. For instance, although Jews do not indulge in heavy drinking, they have a deep-rooted enchantment with gambling as they manage to survive as a small minority community in hostile surroundings. More comprehensively, Bernard Barber (1967) attempted a functional definition of drugs. Among various possible benefits from drug use, he identified aesthetic, aphrodisiac, ego-disrupting, ideological, political, psychological support, religious, research, social control, therapeutic, war, and other conflict functions.

In recent research, there are still studies showing the positive functions of substances and substance use. Klaus Makela and Heli Mustonen (2000) examined drinking behavior in relation to gender and age. Among their interview subjects, women more commonly reported that drinking had helped them to sort out interpersonal problems at home or in the workplace, feel more optimistic about life, and express their feelings. Men more commonly reported that drinking had helped them to be funnier and wittier, and to get closer to the opposite sex. From a developmental perspective, Peter Franzkowiak (1987) compared risk taking to task performing in adolescent development. He noted that smoking and alcohol consumption help adolescents acquire risk-related expertise and competence to fulfill specific developmental tasks and to develop a healthy lifestyle later in their life. At the system level, Kevin Brain, Howard Parker, and Tom Carnwath (2000) analogized substances to consumer goods in the marketplace. Following youth in their self-perception of licit and illicit drug use as functional consumption behavior, they provided an "appreciative" analysis of what, where, and why youth drink in the era of postmodernity when the drink industry becomes ever innovative and aggressive in its marketing of strong, smooth-tasting, image-laden designer drinks, including alcopops. Mark Chapin (1994) applied functional conflict theory to the interactional relationships between the alcoholic beverage industry and the alcoholism treatment industry. He found that the conflicts of interest between the beverage and treatment industries not only are functional for both groups, but also serve the interests of the larger culture.

THEORETICAL FRAMEWORK

Theory begins with facts. The fact is simple and straightforward. Substance use and abuse have been in company with human beings and their survival in nature, as well as their civilizations from society to society, for a long time. It is historically discriminative and logically implausible to just view substance and substance use as marginal, random, deviant, and irrational side products of a generally substantive, consistent, normal, and rational human evolutionary process.

Definition

The functionalist perspective has been marked by its conventional approach or conservative agenda to the study of conforming practices. Applied to substance use, however, it represents a reversal of the conventional or conservative attitude toward the issue. In fact, it sounds far more than liberal when it assumes and is poised to explore various functions substance use serves for individuals and larger economic, political, cultural, and social systems. A more theoretical, systemic, or epistemological portrayal does not seem to dim much of its unconventional overtone or overture when the functionalist perspective is defined as an approach that examines substance and substance use as prevalent and persistent social phenomena, as functional and integral parts of human life, and as necessary and universal elements in natural adaptation and cultural creation by mankind.

No matter how it sounds to the general public, the functionalist perspective looks for every function that substance use contributes to human beings and their social life. Functions are broadly perceived as beneficial, facilitative, or promotional to specific mental or physical activities in terms of frequency, intensity, duration, performance, or result, as well as to specific social processes or institutions with respect to scale, scope, maintenance, effectiveness, efficiency, and consequence. The functionalist perspective will surely shed critical light on and offer unique insights about substance, substance use, and substance users as it attempts to pull the whole issue out of the attic and garret of the socially negative.

Theoretical Image

Human beings are rational beings. Social life is governed by rule and logic. If something exists among human beings and persists in social life from place to place and from time to time, it must have served, be serving, or be about to serve some purposes, either for some parts or for a whole system, either for now or the future, and either for some obvious or underlying reasons. As prevalent and persistent as any other basic human activities, such as food intake, illness, deviance, and artistic creation, substance use must fulfill some more serious, meaningful, and substantive functions other than what is usually expected from wasteful, harmful, or nonpurposive foul plays.

Beginning with substances, there are naturally grown and man-made subtypes. Natural substances grow in specific climates, seasons, or soils. As part of a larger ecosystem, they depend upon and make particular contributions to the environment. When they are identified by human beings as usable substances, they forge a special relationship with one of the species in nature. They are cultivated, harvested, and processed by human beings, giving the species the chance to learn about, as well as the opportunity to strengthen bonds with, nature. Adaptation by human beings improves as they accumulate knowledge about and fine-tune interdependence with various substances in the environment. For example, growing the crop of a substance, processing and preserving harvests, and extracting effective elements from raw materials provide people with needs and motivations to study soils and seasonal changes, develop irrigation systems, invent tools and equipment, and sharpen their management and technical skills. Man-made substances result from a human command and manipulation of physical and chemical properties of various natural substances. Beyond specific utilities they offer for human life, they provide sites for intellectual exercise, embody human intelligence and creativity, and symbolize human triumph over natural limitations and restraints. For example, human beings synthesize a substance that never exists in nature to cure a disease, to change a physical condition, or to modify a mental state.

Substance use, as a human activity, allows people to create, change, convey, and exchange feelings and things in their life. Individuals use substances because substances help them pass time, ease nervousness, reduce anxiety, alleviate pain, clear up thinking, enhance work performance, express emotional sentiments, symbolize status, or entertain themselves. For example, smokers smoke and stay calm, instead of staring at something, running to the restroom, stretching around, or continually washing their hands, when they are anxiously waiting for something. One shows the world how free, relaxing, or self-entertaining he is after leaving his political office when he appears in a photograph holding a smoking cigar on the golf course. Groups use substances because substances assist them to run collective activities, conduct business, maintain discipline and solidarity, or signify group philosophy and commitment. For example, alcohol keeps an organizational gathering going with necessary color and vividness. Cigars, cigarettes, and swirling smoke in a meeting room demonstrate the level of seriousness participants have toward their business interests. Members of a drug use club brave police detection and arrest to show their firm belief in the nonharmfulness of a controlled substance as well as their strong rejection of the injustice that has been waged by the government against its use. Finally, society bears with, tolerates, accommodates, or connives at substance use because it diverts social tension, keeps a portion of the population busy or prevents them from making other more serious trouble, alerts people about moral decay, or fuels economy. In small drug-supply countries, for instance, drug cultivation and trade serve to provide a major source of income for the whole economy. Even in large drug-demand nations, drug distribution and dealing still serve to relieve the state from an otherwise heavier burden of social welfare.

Substance users live and interact with all other members of society. In a variety of roles and positions, they make life and society challenging, eventful, and interesting. First, substance users are consumers, feeding the beverage industry, the service industry, the tobacco industry, and the underground drug economy. Second, they are entertainers, making life easy and fun for people at formal and informal gatherings. Third, they are adventurers, testing the endurance of the human body and the elasticity of the human mind. Fourth, they are revolutionaries, challenging the rationality of cultural norm, law, and social custom. Fifth, they are clients, maintaining the professions of care, help, and counseling. Finally, they are patients, providing cases and conditions for scientific experimentation in science and medicine.

Across societies, substance and substance use bring different cultures, populations, economies, and countries together through exchange, interaction, trade, alliance, and understanding. In cultural exchange and people-to-people interaction, substance and substance use serve as both a common language and a specific symbol. As a common language, they engage people in greeting, conversation, and business or nonbusiness dealings. At a bus stop outside an international airport, two strangers may get into some informal interaction by one borrowing a cigarette or a cigarette lighter from the other even though they do not speak each other's language. A foreign guest may automatically take it as a gesture of welcome when he or she is treated with a local brew by his or her host or hostess. As a specific symbol, substance and substance use provide simple means, terms, or clues for people to identify and treat each other. For a long time, opium and opium dens offered Westerners a general image about the Chinese following the Opium War in 1839–1842. Now as vodka and rocky-feeling spirits provide a sketchy impression about the Russians and the Russian struggle toward democracy, Coca-Cola and polydrug use seem to inspire or fuel a widespread sensation about or distaste for Americans and the American lifestyle by many people around the world.

In trade and political maneuvering, substance and substance use create opportunities, conditions, or excuses for market expansion, brand-name dominance, military intervention, and political alliance. Wines take French exports to societies in both Western and Eastern, both Northern and Southern, hemispheres. Beer leads Germans, Hollanders, and their manufacturing and service products to the heartland of developed countries, as well as the frontier of developing economies. Vodka is one of the most recognizable Russian consumer goods to appear in Western liquor stores and supermarkets. Tobacco represents a leading element in America's multifront corporate expansion into various segments of the world economy. Vineyards, wineries, breweries, tobacco fields, cigarette factories, and various specially prepared alcoholic or psychoactive substances serve their producing or processing localities as tourist attractions, flagship products, or trademark heritages. In the underground drug market, marijuana, heroin, and cocaine bring their respective growing regions specific pricing or name-brand statuses. Politically, the United States and some of its Western allies often use drug eradication as a reason to intervene in military, law enforcement, and other domestic affairs in various countries, especially small and medium-sized countries. In the meantime, peasants, local communities, and national governments in many drug-supplying and -transporting regions tend to bet on drugs and drug-associated problems to gain attention, secure aid, and improve material conditions from governmental agencies or international sources, such as the United Nations and drug-destination countries.

Through history, substance and substance use serve as sites, vehicles, or institutions to socialize the young, to preserve the valuable, and to advance the desirable. Knowledge expands, skills sharpen, and craftsmanship improves from generation to generation when people attempt to grow a substance in a harsh climate or unfavorable soil conditions, expand production or raise output of a substance, cultivate a substance for the best possible quality, preserve and process harvests of a substance, extract effective elements of a substance from raw materials, and transport a substance in varying forms. Within specific cultural, communal, and familial settings, parents may pass on to their children a fine tradition of diligence, thrift, calculation, and survival when they teach them how to maintain and manage the family's tobacco field, vineyard, brewery, liquor store, bar, or other substance-related business. Villagers may reinforce and perpetuate a social custom of fear, respect, and allegiance from the young to the old, from the junior to the senior, and from the poor to the rich when they give and receive toasts at the village's ceremonial events. In some rural areas of China, while the most senior, powerful, or respectable person may feel free to command a toast for anyone at the dinner table, other participants are supposed to offer individual toasts to all those who are more senior, powerful, or respectable than themselves. From culture to culture, it is common that substances, mainly alcohol and tobacco, are used to initiate the young, to mark major rites of passage in life, and to symbolize social values pertaining to authority, social order, and genealogical hierarchy.

Theoretical Components

To understand various possible functions substance serves for users, substance users serve for specific groups, and substance use serves for society, the functionalist perspective focuses on six components in its theoretical analysis.

Function versus Dysfunction

In the war on drugs, political speeches, ideological propaganda, and prevention campaigns, attention has been put on the dysfunction of substance, substance use, and substance user to social order and various institutional establishments. By making a distinction between function and dysfunction, the functionalist perspective attempts to clarify two important points at issue.

One is the subject to whom substance, substance use, and substance user appear to be functional or dysfunctional. Subject variably refers to individuals and specific physical or mental activities within an individual, groups and specific sides or individuals within a group, as well as societies and specific institutions within a society. While to some subjects substance use is dysfunctional, it may well be functional to other subjects. For example, smoking causes coughing, chronic disease, and lung cancer in some individuals while it stimulates intellectual creativity and regulates daily routines for others. English philosopher and mathematician Bertrand

Russell was a heavy smoker. Smoking literally saved his life when he survived a plane crash because he was sitting in the smoking compartment, which was left undamaged. He died at the age of ninety-eight. Within particular subjects, while substance intake is dysfunctional to some body or mind mechanisms, it may be functional to other physical or mental dynamics. For example, marijuana alleviates pain although it causes munching and mellowness, which may lead to obesity and unnecessary withdrawal from productive social engagement. Among groups of subjects, function or dysfunction is not only affected by natural properties pertaining to a substance or substance user, but also defined by individual or social attitudes, positions, and contexts regarding the substance and its users. For example, children's use of inhalants may be considered dysfunctional by parents as it challenges parental discipline, erodes family morality, and drains household finances. But by children themselves, it may be taken as something functional in relieving stress, creating excitement, and promoting friendship.

The other point is the relativity of both function and dysfunction. Function is not absolute, nor is dysfunction. From the past to the present and from the present to the future, function may change in degree, cease to exist, or revert to dysfunction. Across space, function may vary in intensity, vanish from existence, or switch to dysfunction. By different criteria, function or dysfunction may appear in various scales, forms, and utilities from one extreme, through the middle range, to the other extreme. For example, drinking rejuvenates the atmosphere at a party when people talk, dance, and socialize with each other. It could lead to traffic accidents on the road when the same group of people drive home from the party. Heroine use serves to relieve pain from hard labor for some southeast Asians in their remote mountain villages. It makes them drug addicts, welfare dependents, and treatment targets when they migrate to the United States and cluster in urban enclaves. Time, location, and frame of reference can singly or jointly turn the sides of a same act back and forth from function to dysfunction, even for the same group of actors.

Manifest versus Latent Functions

Manifest functions are those consequences intended, expected, or recognized by the actor or audience from an act. Latent functions, in contrast, are unintended, unexpected, or unrecognized consequences of an act by the actor or the audience. As far as substance use is concerned, manifest functions may include pain relieving, mind refreshing, body revitalizing, excitement creating, intelligence enhancing, or resentment expressing. Latent functions, on the other hand, may include the individual gaining attention and status, the group strengthening coherence and solidarity, and the society unleashing strain and tension.

In the concrete, substances manifest their functions as crops to grow, products to process, merchandise to trade, objects to learn, and things to use. When people deal with a substance, the substance latently serves as a reason or site for people to expand knowledge; sharpen skills; invent tools, production procedures, or equipment; and develop treatment methods or modalities. For example, the identification of maintenance programs in drug treatment can be seen as a latent function of heroine abuse. Similarly, substance use manifests its functions for users as pain alleviation, mind stimulation, mood tranquilization, or performance enhancement. In latent form, users gain attention or enhance their status while engaging in conspicuous or substantive use of substances. For example, an intravenous drug user injects drugs to maintain his or her physical condition under the situation of addiction. To awould-be intravenous drug user, he or she may serve as an ultimate model of courage, toughness, and endurance. To treatment and law enforcement officers, he or she may exist as a challenge or opportunity for creative and effective intervention. Finally, substance users manifest their functions to society as consumers, customers, clients, innovators, fashioners, or messengers. As society faces substance users in various situations, it may engage itself in collective reflection and action upon human liability and susceptibility in both the natural and social environments. In other words, while substance users manifestly keep society on its toes with practical issues, they latently motivate people to contemplate the nature, purpose, and destiny of their increasingly materialistic life. For example, people learn from substance users about the power of addiction. They may decide to fight drug abuse through moral resort, a change of behavior, or the power of an effective medicine.

Material versus Moral Functions

Material function generally refers to any consequence substance use may cause in body, body appearance and function, resource, and resource exchange and distribution. It may fall under both manifest and latent functions. As far as body is concerned, substance use may help one allay pain, fight depression, and manage stress. It may help him or her stay active, calm, or alert on dangerous or important duty. It may serve him or her as an activity to kill time, an igniter to start work, a breaker to take rest, a marker to identify important issues or events, or a regulator to follow routine. For instance, in total institutions where people are pushed to a halt or minimum in their bodily activity, they may use smoking and drug taking just to keep their body operational. In the cold weather, people take alcoholic drinks to keep warm. Smokers smoke cigarettes or pipes to wake up, break away from work, fall asleep, and follow their daily schedule. Coffee break is standard terminology in white-collar work settings.

Individual habits, idiosyncracies, and situations abound regarding substance use as intentionally functional: "I drink a cup of tea before I work"; "I take a specially prepared herb soup one week before I participate in a sport competition"; "I feel uncomfortable if I eat a hamburger without a glass of iced Coke"; "I drink wine when I eat meat"; "I feel restful when I smoke opium after a long, hard day of labor in the field"; "I keep my erection strong and long when I take 'meth'"; or "I take speed when I sleep on the street."

In terms of resource, substance and substance use may serve as material means to draw people and resources into a community, a region, or a country. On the one hand, licit or illicit substance dealing and dealers bring in money, maintaining an on-the-ground or underground economy involving production, processing, trade, transportation, communication, and financial service. Local farmers, manual laborers, merchants, technicians, financiers, or gang leaders thrive or survive on the substance-related economic activities. On the other hand, substance regulation, substance use control, and substance user treatment keep the presence of politicians, law enforcement officials, social service personnel, and treatment professionals in the scene surrounding substance and its use. Government assistance, social welfare, and private contributions flow in, making local residents attended to and cared for in many aspects of their life. In a latent form, substance use redistributes social wealth that was originally distributed to the disadvantage of the poor, the weak, the powerless, or the underrepresented. For instance, wealthy substance users spend money on substances, sending part of their wealth back to growers, dealers, or petty shopkeepers who are usually exploited in the whole economic system. From a global point of view, Western societies harvest tremendous economic benefits when they export technology and equipment to and import labor-intensive consumer goods from developing countries. Rampant substance use and abuse in Western societies, in a sense, serve to repatriate some of the economic benefits they garner from around the world through export-import as well as corporate expansion, back to their original sources, specifically some drug-supply countries as representative recipients.

Compared to material function, moral function includes any consequence substance use has on the mind, emotion, morality, social norm, and cultural standard. At the individual level, substance use may change mood, modify feelings, and make life cheerful and enjoyable. It may create illusion, intensify some sentiments, and take life to a transcendental latitude. It may inactivate conventional prohibition, loosen moral restraints, and lead one to a new world of "do and don't." In a nutshell, substance use may serve individuals as an eye opener to see different perspectives, an adventurer to explore and expand the vast landscape of the mind, and a reformer to experiment with new rules and ways of life. With respect to social norm, no matter whether it is considered to be right or wrong, substance use exists as a site, occasion, or thing for people to make judgments, learn lessons, educate the young, and take appropriate actions. Regarding cultural standards, substance use creates contexts and issues for people to debate and negotiate on tolerance versus intolerance, maintenance versus treatment, and accommodation versus eradication. For example, socially defined licit substance use is maintained as an institutional practice while being questioned as a health hazard. Individuals take use as a sign or symbol of autonomy, maturity, responsibility, importance, power, or status. Socially defined illicit substance use is controlled as a moral deviance while being admired by some as a breakthrough from tradition or a step forward into the future. Individuals remain divided on the meaning of use. They either look upon it as a protest against the status quo and a harbinger of new life, or look down upon it as an indication of moral decline and a turn to human regression. In abstract or universalistic terms, as stated by classic functionalists, substance use sets moral boundaries, clarifies sentiments, and unites people in their respective camps.

Short-Term versus Long-Term Functions

An important dimension to the effect of substance use is time. Short-term functions are effects users experience during and not long after use. Applying the three distinctions made above, short-term effects are more likely to be functions than dysfunctions, manifest than latent functions, and material than moral functions. For instance, most users experiment with a substance because they are interested in its immediate effects. They would feel disappointed and hence change their learned view about the substance if they did not receive some of the instant body or mood reactions to it: "See, it does not make me laugh, it does not make me light-headed, it does not take me to the kind of dream trip you guys claim." In the sense that users expect to experience all or some of its effects during and after the use of a substance, every effect expected from the substance, no matter whether it is positive or negative, favorable or unfavorable, qualifies as a short-term function. In other words, feeling relaxed and a need for munchies serve marijuana users not only as an ongoing sign of the effectiveness of the drug taken, but also as an introductory signal of the ultimate mellowness expected from marijuana. Similarly to any other drug, users are likely to question or feel uneasy about the substance taken if they do not experience bitterness, a feeling of rash, a cramp, accelerated heartbeats, watery eyes, a running nose, or a red face as commonly expected from its initial intake.

Long-term functions include effects users accumulate on their body and mind though continuous exposure to a substance. If short-term effects are functional because they are intended and expected, various long-term functions can be hazardous because they are unintended and unexpected. For instance, smokers may rely upon smoking to regulate their mood and daily routine. Staying in the smoking section of a room may happen to save a smoker's life from an accident. But in the long run, smokers may have to deal with some chronic illness in their respiratory system, and possibly face a final judgment on life and death, lung cancer, as in the case of many smokers. There are, however, possible long-term benefits from substance use as well. Speculatively, exposures to different substances may exercise and train the human body and mind in substance accommodation, tolerance, endurance, or adaptation. Scientifically, reports are forthcoming with regard to the functionality of wine, beer, and other substances to human health and longevity in the form of long-term and moderate use.

Beyond individual users, short-term versus long-term functions can be analyzed on substances as well as substance use and users in society. For instance, growing, processing, or synthesizing a substance may create jobs, promote trade, and facilitate research in particular periods and locales. In the long run, it may increase scientific knowledge, diversify foods and medicine, or maintain balance in the ecosystem. Regarding substance use and users in society, it keeps people alert on various social problems they face and unites people behind their concerted effort against moral decay when it develops into an epidemic. Some substance users may challenge medical professionals with an opportunity to develop new treatment and medicine as they emerge with unique symptoms or physical conditions from long, multiple use. In a long-term perspective, substance use teaches people about life, human nature, and all the contradictions and predicaments associated with human life.

Peripheral versus Core Functions

From a medical as well as social control point of view, it might be useful to make a distinction between peripheral and core functions for substance and substance use. Peripheral functions are effects a substance causes in particular areas, periods of time, or on specific activities of a system that remain local, regional, marginal, or relatively unimportant in comparison to the whole system and the grand or ultimate goal of the system. For instance, opioid drugs, while acting on the central nervous system, produce analgesia, a sense of tranquility, a decreased sense of apprehension, and a suppression of the cough reflex. They slow passage of food in the stomach and in small and large intestines while acting on the gastrointestinal system. They increase sphincter tone and decrease the voiding reflexes while acting on the bladder (Jaffe 1992). However, in the whole physiological system of an opiate drug user, all these different effects, no mater how medically functional they each appear to be, become marginal, peripheral, and even irrelevant to the severe symptoms of narcotic addiction. Similarly, in a diverse social system, substance use may be entertaining, facilitative of group coherence, or expressive of individual or group sentiments in a particular subculture or among a specific segment of the population. But all these group-based functions may end up to be just an insignificant episode, if not a nuisance, in the whole social drama, let alone when society is poised to fight substance use and abuse as a rampant social problem.

Core functions revolve around major effects substance use has on a system and its general goal or activity. Specific effects substance use causes in a particular part of the system may also qualify as core functions when that part is highlighted as the center of attention. For instance, when sex and sex organ are focused, sexual excitation and spontaneous ejaculation without direct genital stimulation in particular may become core functions of cocaine use (Gold 1992). Except those in relative terms, core functions in general terms include all systemwide effects a substance is known to have on the human organism. For example, amphetamines and other stimulants manifest their central effects in neurochemical and electro-physiological systems. Benzodiazepines and barbiturates have sedative, antipanic, anticonvulsant, analgesic, and hypnotic functions. Hallucinogens cause somatic, perceptual, and psychic effects. Perceptual effects, such as altered visual sense and change in hearing, and psychic effects, such as dreamlike feelings and change in mood, are core functions hallucinogen users actively seek in their use experience. In the larger social system, since substance use has been treated negatively as a social problem, most core functions can be identified only in abstract or latent form. For example, substance use serves to remind people about social inequality and human susceptibility. It unites people in their joint fight against moral decline. There are, however, concrete or manifest core functions from substance use as well. Some obvious functions are: substance use stimulates the economy, recharges politics, rejuvenates ideological debates, and redistributes social wealth across the population.

Alternative Functions

The functionalist theory not only identifies functional prerequisites, or "preconditions functionally necessary for a society" (Merton 1957: 87), but also functional alternatives, or substitutes that perform the same task for a given social structure or institution. As far as substance use is concerned, does it serve as a functional alternative for some individual acts, social institutions, or cultural practices? What are those individual acts, social institutions, or cultural practices? What alternative functions does it substitute for them specifically?

At the individual level, anxiety, depression, anger, and emotional blast are common human feelings and expressions. Instead of yelling, screaming, kicking stuff, taking a scapegoat, or remaining nervous, restless, fearful, lonely, scared, and painful, one may drink a beer, smoke a cigarette, or take some drugs to calm himself down or to nullify his inner impulse toward self-suppression or expression. Substance use therefore serves as a functional alternative to drastic physical and mental actions. In society, complaint, protest, rebellion, and crime are universal and consistent phenomena. While it is normally believed that drug abuse leads to crime, it is logically and theoretically plausible that substance use substitutes for crime and other more violent, perversive, or harmful forms of antisocial behavior. It is hence possibly true that crime and other more serious social offenses would have occurred at a more alarmingly high rate had there been no substance use and abuse. Across cultures, misunderstanding, conflict, confrontation, and war take place from time to time. Throughout history, substance used to occasionally serve as a bloodless alternative for one nation to conquer, disable, or tranquilize another. In the eyes of many Chinese, opium was just another weapon used by Western imperialists in the invasion into their age-old civilizations. In the contemporary globalized world economy, licit and illicit substances seem to have more alternative functions to play in many more dimensions. For some nationalist radicals, substances symbolize their nation's power to counteract the omnipresent dominance of Western capitalist countries: "We too have something to break into your society and put you on the defense at home." In trade, they substitute conventional goods to keep export or import in relative balance. In politics, they act as alternatives to diplomacy, power, and military advantage for nations to gain attention, importance, and influence in the world.

In other words, substance and substance use, if they themselves are evils, still provide alternatives to some even greater and more devastating evils that individuals, groups, and societies have to deal with in their survivals.

Theoretical Applications

From a functionalist point of view, it is always possible and heuristic to identify and explore both practical utilities and moralistic functions for substances, substance use, and substance users.

Beginning with substance, what natural properties does a particular substance have to make it selected by human beings from millions of plant or animal products in their living environment? Is it selected for medical use, for recreational purpose, or as a nutritional, flavoring, or coloring ingredient in food? What specific growing, synthesizing, processing, preserving, or packaging procedures or techniques have been developed or modified to raise its productivity, purify its quality, sharpen its effect, change its form, or boost its price from place to place as well as over time? Has it grown into larger political, economic, social, and cultural systems, becoming an enemy target, a production or trade item, an expression of difference, or a symbol of status? What essential characteristics does it have to keep it on and off public attention? For example, alcohol has been in the picture of recorded human life for a long time. With a wide range of use from industry, recreation, medicine, and household to personal consumption, alcohol is well integrated in the production and trade system, as well as in culture, diplomacy, and politics in many societies around the world.

Regarding substance use, does it alleviate pain for users? Does it help them recover from injury or some physical ailments? Does it improve inner experience for users? Does it help them deal with stress, depression, or other ill feelings? Does it create different perceptions, moods, or abilities for users? Does it help them function faster, smarter, or with higher efficiency and productivity on job duty or in life routine? For groups and societies, what does substance use say about and suggest to them? Does it indicate dissatisfaction, dissent, or rebellion from the populace? Does it convey problems inherent in morality, law, and social structure? Does it call for change in cultural practice, social institution, and political control? More directly to the advantage of a group or society, does substance use ease tension, divert conflict, and prevent serious deviations? Does it create and maintain jobs? Does it promote trade? Does it facilitate exchange and interaction within and among groups? Does it bring people together in unity and solidarity? For instance, drug abuse triggers the drug war. The drug war connects politicians to the populace, law enforcement officers to local residents, and middle-class professionals to lower-class drunkards and addicts, in the seemingly united crusade against drug abuse, despite their respective differences. Drug abuse is also the primary reason why thousands of jobs are created and maintained in law, criminal justice, treatment, and social service.

With respect to users, what unique experiences do they have to prompt them to use a substance? What specific encounter do they run into with a substance? What do they say or demonstrate about each episode, stage, or symptom they pass through in their relation with a substance? Physically, do substance users serve as sites for scientific observation and medical research? Mentally, are they messengers of psychological change or targets of psychiatric evaluation and treatment? In the sense that substance users verbally and nonverbally express what they feel before, during, and after substance use, they diversify and expand the whole human experience as it is known to the majority. For instance, if a substance instantly changes human feelings from despair to joy, only a user of the substance can tell or show that the substance does indeed have that special power and that despair is indeed replaceable by joy in the twinkling of an eye. In addition to what they speak and illustrate about human reactions toward substance and substance use, do substance users act as a source of concern, bringing siblings, parents, relatives, friends, neighbors, or colleagues together in a family, a work organization, or a community? Do they change family and community perceptions and attitudes about substance, substance use, substance users, and generally people in need? To the larger social system, what relevance and significance do substance users have? Are they vital consumers? Are they messengers of social change? Or are they just troublemakers whose only positive function is to keep people alert and busy?

Empirical Tests

Given the general climate and sentiment about substance use and abuse, empirical research in the perspective of functionalism requires not only courage to do what not everyone does, but also critical thinking skills to explore what not everyone recognizes.

Case studies follow individual substances or users. Functions of a substance can be documented in relation to a variety of factors. For example, some of its functions may be specific to where it is produced, how it is processed, what purity it has in a specific form, and whether it is used with some other supplements. Some of its functions may be manifested only in particular areas of the body on which it acts or particular types of mind functions upon which it impacts. It is also interesting to ascertain what side effects it has, what dosage is usually required to achieve a minimal, medium, or maximal result, and what interactive substances it has to counteract to preserve, modify, or reinforce its own effects. For individual users, studies may detail how they perceive functions or dysfunctions of a particular substance, how they adjust themselves to the widely known effects of a substance, whether an experienced function is accidental, developmental, gradual, or long-lasting, and what effort they make to manage the actual function or dysfunction of their substance use so that they remain functional on their ordinary duty in work and life. A lot can be learned about a substance and specific modes of use by studying cases in which use becomes functional to normal body and mind activities, and users never lose control over their habit.

If case studies are geared to uncover unique functions of particular substances among specific users, survey research is equipped to identify common effects of a substance experienced by a sizable group of users through some widely recognized modes of use. A function or dysfunction of a substance becomes recognized and established only when it is similarly experienced and reported by most of its users. For existing substances, survey research verifies their functions or dysfunctions through known routes of administration or new forms of consumption. For emerging substances, it reveals how positive or negative effects occur after varying frequency, intensity, or method of use and abuse. It is interesting to note that most descriptive features about a substance, as recorded in the literature, are based upon numerous user reports gathered through survey or interview, although each of those features pertains only to the particular case of the substance. For example, a dream trip effect of a hallucinogen becomes known and validated when user after user share their similar stories about it.

Experimental studies involve observation and measurement in both laboratories and natural settings. In laboratories, animals and human subjects may be used to ascertain if different dosages of a substance on a varying schedule result in specific physical or mental reactions. Does it increase or decrease heartbeat, blood flow, skin temperature, mobile skill, alertness, or violent behavior? Does a substance-induced change in one region or part of the body positively or negatively affect the function of the whole organism? Why do some consequences from substance use become functional while others turn dysfunctional? Is there an interactive agent that mediates the effect of the substance? In natural settings, quasi-experimental designs provide an opportunity to verify if personal perception and attitudes counteract or modify a substance's natural effect and make its use functional or dysfunctional in particular situations. For instance, meaningful comparisons can be made between a group with exposure and a group without exposure to some critical subcultural messages, to see if justification or glamorization about a controlled substance in the user subculture makes users experience more of the substance's positive effects. Similarly, useful information can be obtained to substantiate if prevention and health education make a difference in individual experience with a substance, through a quasi-experimental study in which one group is educated only about the benefit of the substance and the other is taught only about the harm of the substance.

POLICY IMPLICATIONS

With the spotlight long having been on the negative effects of substance use and abuse, some attention to and knowledge of their positive functions can have critical impacts on policy and action.

Public Health

Medical diagnosis and treatment are based upon scientific research. Doctors and other health professionals are supposed to explore and know all possible effects, both positive and negative, of commonly used and abused substances, regardless of their personal ideology and social value orientations. However, since most funding is provided to study the harmful aspect of substance use and abuse, the whole health community seems to heavily lean toward addiction, dependency, disorder, malfunction, and other adverse syndromes resultant from abuse, not only in their own investigation but also in their communications with the general public.

Under the functionalist perspective, health professionals can take a balanced approach toward substance use and abuse. While focusing on abuse, they may explore the full range of use in terms of purity, dosage, scheduling, personal adaptation, and counteragent. Information about both benefits and harms of a substance is indiscriminately gathered and made available to the public so that people can make their own decision about use or nonuse. While concentrating on users or abusers as patients in need of help, health professionals may view them as valuable research subjects from whom they indispensably benefit in advancing medical knowledge and strengthening treatment protocols. On a more subtle level, they may regard their substance use or abuse clients as likable and respectable neighbors and friends from whom they learn about various human conditions and needs.

Social Control

With their concrete duties of catching, sentencing, or guarding drug dealers, users, and troublemakers, social control agents probably do not have any time to ponder how their enemy targets keep their profession, making them continuously modernize their equipment, update their facility, and sharpen their job skills. Nor do they possibly have any leisure to appreciate how their control subjects put the general public on defensive alert so that they can handily rely upon some concerted cooperation and support from local residents, business leaders, and politicians in their prevention and intervention operations.

While the functionalist perspective reminds social control agents to reflect upon the function of substance use and users in abstract terms, it provides them concrete warnings in various areas and occasions of their jobs as well. When law enforcement officials spot marijuana plants or bust loads of cocaine, they do not destroy them because they know marijuana or cocaine itself is not an enemy and it instead can be saved for functional use in recreation or medical treatment. When judges preside over a case on drug dealing, possession, or use, they do not presumptively deliver judgment and impose sanction because they know drug activity itself is not a sin and it instead may be functional to economy, trade, health, or personal welfare. When prison guards see inmates smoke cigarettes or use drugs, they do not react with a crackdown because they know smoking or using drugs itself is not a problem and it instead may function to keep inmates quiet and the total institution under control. It is obvious that all these rational reactions in recognition of the function of substance use and users will not occur until significant change takes place in the law and social control. Hopefully, insights from the functionalist perspective will gradually influence social control agents and the general populace so that change comes along eventually.

Life and Community

Parents, siblings, relatives, friends, and local residents probably have difficulty comprehending any function of substance use and abuse when they see their loved ones, friends, or neighbors struggling with addiction, dealing drugs, running from the police, or being locked up for drug-related offenses. In fact, when they live under fear and compromise the quality of life because drug dealers compete for turf and drug users seek money through prostitution or by illegal means in their neighborhood, people naturally blame drugs and drug use for everything negative they may be able to think of.

Despite immediate and commonsensical reactions, people in the long run will be able to go beyond their firsthand experience and to evaluate a phenomenon in a larger context as well as in a more philosophical sense. Life is, after all, a multilayered and multifaceted prism. The meaning of life lies in not only content, the positive, the concrete, and the immediate, but also form, the negative, the abstract, and the remote. Substances may first appear to be health hazards but may also afford life and the community with choices and alternatives. Substance use may first appear to be a nuisance but may also enrich life and the neighborhood with different activities and lifestyles. Substance users may first appear to be troublemakers but may also serve as vital clients or customers. In a family, for example, one member's experience with a substance may educate the whole family about human susceptibility, liability, sympathy, care, tolerance, and forgiveness. It may thus make all other family members more balanced persons, both morally and emotionally. In a community, likewise, people may become more compassionate, objective, and systematic in their world outlook when they realize substance use and users may remind them of some more fundamental problems, may suggest solutions or alternatives, and may bring them together in collective actions.

Work and Organization

At present, functions of substance and substance use in work and organizational settings are manifested in five major areas: (a) steroids and some stimulants enhance performance in sports and competition; (b) some substances counteract hazardous conditions or possible dangers faced by workers and soldiers; (c) drug testing may assist employers to screen out potentially troublesome employees; (d) an employer assistant program in substance use and abuse may serve as an image builder and beautifier; and (e) a coffee lounge, smoking area, or on- or off-site bar provided for employees may work for a company as the motivator for employee loyalty and dedication.

With insights from the functionalist perspective, employment organizations may take a more active, open, and accommodating approach toward substance use and abuse among their employees. First, they may feel obligated to study their specific work and working conditions to see if those conditions prompt functional or dysfunctional use of a substance. Second, they may actively explore functions of existing and new substances to see if some of them act to enhance job performance, relieve work-related pain and stress, counteract job-induced side effects, or prevent likely dangers and injuries. Third, they may assess their drug testing, employer assistance, and other substance-related programs as part of the whole employee benefit and service package to see if they may use each of them to improve employee service, raise employee morale, and forge collective solidarity with the majority of employees. Fourth, employment organizations may take substance use and abuse as an opportunity to engage in the community. They may offer their professional knowledge and financial resources, making themselves a valuable establishment in the neighborhood. Finally, confronting substance use and abuse by its employees and reaching out to the community in substance-related service may help an organization realize its broader connection to and larger role in society. It may thus become a more responsible and functional unit in social process.

In all, the functionalist perspective begins with common and conventional beliefs: human beings are rational—if they do something, that something must serve them a purpose; and social institutions are functional—if they occur and continue over time and from place to place, they must play some part in the larger social structure and broader social process. On the matter of substance use and abuse, however, the functionalist perspective obviously leads to uncommon and unconventional statements: people produce and use substances with some purposes; substance use exists and persists for some reasons; and substance users fit into society and fulfill some functions for it.

Aside from the conventional versus unconventional contrast or conservative versus liberal confrontation, the functionalist perspective as a mere scientific approach focuses on effects or consequences that substance, substance use, and substance user have for their respective carriers, subjects, groups, or contexts. In the concrete sense, functions or positive effects may range from pain alleviation, symptom management, stress control, socializing, exchange, trade activities, and service provision, to job creation. Dysfunctions or negative consequences may involve dependency, withdrawal syndrome, social vice, crime, black market, waste of social resources, and drain on the taxpayers' money. On an abstract level, the functionalist perspective explores how substance may improve human adaptation to nature, how substance use and abuse may act as a substitute for more serious deviance and even crime in a society, and how substance users may serve their group, culture, and historical era as messengers of critical issues or innovators of alternative lifestyles.

With the functionalist perspective, substance, substance use, and substance users can be placed in a broader time frame and a larger spatial context so that their latent, long-term, moral, and abstract consequences are examined in relation to their manifest, immediate, material, and concrete effects, and their functions or positive contributions are evaluated in balance with their dysfunctions or negative impacts.

—5—

The Rational Choice Perspective

No matter how it appears to be, legal or illegal, healthy or unhealthy, beneficial or harmful, rational or irrational, substance use is chosen by individuals, groups, and societies. Individual human beings possess will and intelligence. Human groupings operate under self-interest and rationality. The choice of substance use therefore must involve a considerable level of reasoning, on the part of users or use groups, over essential variables, such as risk, reward, pain, pleasure, cause, and consequence.

The rational choice perspective centers on human rationality in its effort to understand substance, substance use, and substance users. It examines why a substance is adopted for use, why certain substance use is regulated pertaining to age, gender, or occasion, and how individuals make their choice about use or nonuse, all under the premise of human rationality. While it primarily follows rationality in its normal functioning, the rational choice perspective logically points to the side of irrationality for critical inquiry. For instance, can users make normally rational choices under the influence of drugs? Is there clouded reasoning, twisted rationality, or impaired judgment in the context of addiction? The rational choice perspective also investigates what range of rationality or irrationality a society may exhibit in its reaction to substance use and abuse as a social problem.

SOURCES OF INSPIRATION

The rational choice perspective has roots in the classical school of criminology. The groundwork for classic criminology was laid by Italian social thinker Cesare Beccaria in his 1764 treatise *An Essay on Crimes and*

Punishments. According to Beccaria (1963), humans are rational hedonists who explore and assess available alternatives to maximize pleasure and minimize pain. Assuming that pleasure is gained from a deviating or law-breaking act, punishment ought to be rationally and proportionally meted out to inflict pain in amounts greater than the pleasure achieved from the act. Only when deviant or criminal acts are dealt punishments that are certain, swift, and more severe than the acts themselves can deviants and criminals be deterred from seeking pleasure through those acts. As far as the whole social control system is concerned, Beccaria argued: (a) that only legislators should create laws; (b) that judges should not interpret laws but should only impose punishment in accordance with the law; (c) that laws should be used to maintain social contracts, with equal treatment to all people in the jurisdiction; (d) that punishment should be based on the act, not on the actor; and (e) that it is more desirable to prevent crimes than to punish them.

In Britain, Beccaria's ideas were popularized by philosopher Jeremy Bentham in his writings on utilitarianism. Like Beccaria, Bentham (1967) believed that all human actions are calculated in accordance with their likelihood to produce advantage, pleasure, and happiness and to avoid or prevent mischief, pain, or unhappiness. With respect to law, he argued that laws should produce and support the greatest happiness for the greatest number of people. Regarding punishment, he reasoned that since it is in itself harmful, punishment should be justified only if it promises to prevent greater evil than it creates. Specifically, Bentham prescribed four main objectives for punishment: (a) to prevent all criminal offenses; (b) to convince offenders to commit less serious crimes; (c) to persuade offenders to use no or less force in the commission of crime; and (d) to minimize cost in the social reaction to crime.

Beccaria and Bentham were well embraced in the Western world for their rationalistic views on crime and punishment. In England, criminal law underwent a complete reform between 1820 and 1861. In North America, the Eighth Amendment against cruel and unusual punishment was incorporated into the U.S. Constitution. The most classical application, however, was the famous French Penal Code of 1791. The code was strictly explicit in its attempt "not only to legislate on every crime, but to fix by statute the penalty for each degree of each kind" (Gillin 1945: 229). Because of the code and its overly rigid rationality, a number of neo-classical modifications were explored later on several fronts, including premeditation, circumstance, and mental competence. On the matter of premeditation, should first-time offenders be given more severe punishment because they are freer in will and are less locked in the force of habit? Regarding circumstance, do weather, climate, stress, pressure, and situational factors affect offenders in their choice of crime? And with respect to mental condition, should some deviant actors not be held accountable for their acts by virtue of insanity? The most visible influence of classic criminology, of course, is the construction of the Panopticon, "a mill to grind rogues honest and idle men industrious" (Bentham 1843: 226). Despite ideological ups and downs in rational punishment debates, the centralized control of deviants and criminals in state penitentiaries has since become a standard correctional practice around the world.

Rational choice ideas were brushed aside when positivistic quests for causes of crime took dominance in criminology. It was not until the late 1960s, when "disillusionment sets in about the capacity to fully understand the etiology of crime" and when "reservations are increasingly being expressed about the rehabilitative goals of penal philosophy and correctional practices," that "the basic framework . . . of Beccaria's and Bentham's ideas is slowly infiltrating back into criminological studies" (Sheleff 1981: 3, 6). First, Marvin Wolfgang, Robert Figlio, and Thorsten Sellin (1972) made reference to classical control ideas in their proposed model of rational deterrence. Based upon their finding that most offenders fall out of the pool of delinquents after one or two offenses, they suggest that little should be done with delinquent youth until they arrive at a third offense. In response to their finding that a small group of chronic offenders are responsible for over half of the total number of all offenses recorded for a whole cohort, they propose that the full force of sanction should be reserved for offenders who strike out a third time. Severity of punishment should increase heavily and proportionally for each subsequent offense. People who commit more than a threshold number of offenses should perhaps be locked up forever.

Culminating the revival of classical views on crime and deviance is the publication of *Thinking about Crime* by political scientist James Q. Wilson. Firing at the positivist view that crime is a function of external forces and can therefore be altered by governmental programs, Wilson (1975) argued that control efforts should be focused on deterring would-be offenders and incarcerating known criminals. According to Wilson, most people are neither wicked nor innocent. They are watchful, dissembling, and calculating of their chances. They ponder social reaction to wickedness as a clue to what they might profitably do. If they are convinced that their actions will certainly be met by swift punitive response, only the totally irrational would be willing to engage in crime. On the other hand, if society does not forcefully react to crime, prospective offenders who sit on the fence will get a clear message: crime pays.

Classic criminology, neoclassic modifications, and positivistic rebuttals altogether provide fertile intellectual soil for the development of the contemporary rational choice perspective (Cornish and Clarke 1986). The central tenets of the perspective are: people choose to commit or forgo crime in consideration of both personal and situational factors; personal factors that a reasoning criminal usually weighs in include his or her needs for material gains, thrills, or revenge, his or her criminal skills, and his or her access to legitimate avenues for success; and situational factors that a rational offender evaluates may range from the vulnerability of the target, the location of the operation, the reward of criminal undertaking, and the risk of apprehension, to the severity of punishment. In alignment with routine activities theory, rational choice theory further claims that crime is a product of criminal opportunity. Opportunity opens up when suitable targets, such as corner homes, secluded properties, unlocked cars, open doors, unattended luggage, and access streets into the neighborhood from traffic arteries, become available. It increases when capable guardians, including police officers, vigilant residents, security fences, and household alarms, are absent. Opportunity may also interact with criminal motivation to create various patterns of crime amid specific routine activities in a given environment. For example, urban environments make suitable victims and attractive targets because they gather an enormous collection of consumer goods, commercial establishments, and material utilities. They continually produce and reproduce motivated offenders because they support a highly fluid lifestyle through mass media, advanced means of transportation, and peer networking (Clarke 1995).

Once settling its theoretical assumption that offenders act rationally, the rational choice perspective places its major emphasis on how to practically deal with them. Among various proposed control actions are four main strategies: situational crime prevention, general deterrence, specific deterrence, and incapacitation. Under situational crime prevention, Ronald Clarke and Ross Homel (1997) identify four groups of effective techniques to reduce criminal incidents. Group I focuses on increasing perceived effort through such techniques as target hardening, access control, deflecting offenders, and controlling facilitators. For example, a tough gun control legislation may make it difficult for potential offenders to gain access to guns as crime facilitators. Group II includes entry/exit screening, formal surveillance by security devices or guards, surveillance by employees, and natural surveillance through street lighting. The general intent is to increase perceived risks. Group III involves a reduction of anticipated rewards by way of target removal, identifying property, reducing temptation, and denying benefits. For instance, a gender-neutral telephone list may reduce temptation for telephone harassment on women victims. Finally, Group IV centers on inducing guilt or shame. It includes rule setting, strengthening moral condemnation, controlling disinhibitors, and facilitating compliance. To control or discourage drinking, for example, a drinking age law is put in place to prevent underage alcohol use. Signs like "bloody idiots drink and drive" are attached to the rear bumper of cars to deride and discourage potential violators.

General deterrence is to make potential criminals fear the consequences of crime. If criminals are rational and if they know crime is punished, they will choose not to commit crime. Specific deterrence is to punish known criminals so that they will never repeat their offenses. The reasoning is the same: a rational criminal learns from his or her painful experience with punishment. Three variables critically pertain to the effect of deterrence (Gibbs 1968). They are: certainty, severity, and celerity. Certainty requires that criminals are caught and punished definitely for their lawbreaking behaviors. A person with criminal friends may not fear punishment much if he or she learns from them how easy it is to get away with crime. Severity is about the level of pain, suffering, or threat inflicted or posed by punishment. The stiffer a sanction is, the more effectively it is supposed to deter crime. Celerity refers to the speed with which a sanction is applied to an offender or offense. The swifter it is imposed, the more effective it is to prevent future offense. The three variables are obviously interrelated. The death penalty, the most severe form of punishment, would lose its rigor if it took a considerable portion of an offender's lifetime for him or her to be executed for a capital offense. In addition to certainty, severity, and swiftness, studies also point to other variables, such as perception and informal sanctions, as important influences on penal effectiveness. For example, John Braithwaite (1989) argues that crime control should incorporate reintegrative shaming, by which criminal offenders are made to understand their wrongdoing and shame themselves before they are forgiven and reaccepted by society.

Incapacitation attempts to reduce crime by denying motivated offenders the opportunity to commit it. There are first critical ages during which people are more at risk for criminal offense. If offenders are placed behind bars in their prime crime years, they miss their lifetime opportunity to commit crime and develop a criminal career. There are then a core of chronic offenders who account for a large percentage of crime in society. If they are selectively incarcerated under a "three strikes and you're out" policy or similar measures, they significantly shorten their span of criminal career and contribute fewer offenses to the whole stock of crime (Greenwood 1982). While advocates claim that it leads to actual decline and overall stabilization in some crimes, incapacitation itself causes a number of problems as well. First, it results in a steep increase in the prison population. Second, prison maintenance and management are costly. Third, some offenders are unnecessarily locked up for an unnecessarily long time. Fourth, crowdedness and deteriorating conditions make prisons a fertilizing ground for future criminality. Inmates recidivate and return to prison often because they have prior experiences in incarceration (Wallerstedt 1984). Finally, there are always motivated people to take the place of incarcerated offenders as long as benefits can be made from crime. For example, local gang members may take over a drug market when organized crime leaders are imprisoned.

In the field of substance use and abuse, "the drug of choice" has long become a standard phrase, signifying the importance of individual selection and adaptation in use initiation, experimentation, and habituation with an available pool of substances. Through empirical studies, physicians, clinical researchers, and medical scientists explore the effects of abusable substances on brain reward mechanisms (Gardner 1992). Psychologists relate substance use to personality, individuation, and maturity in an attempt to find differences among users in cognitive style, analytical skill, defense strategy, and other individual choice variables (Mider 1983; Spotts and Shontz 1985; Kerr 1996). From a broader social point of view, researchers make efforts to pin down how economic, cultural, and social forces or interests shape individual choices on substance use and treatment. For example, Robert Agnew (1990) examined National Survey of Youth data and found that individuals commit drug offenses not only due to social pressure, but also because of self-gratification and pleasure. Steinar Andersen and John Berg (1997) followed a sample of substance abusers who were residents of drug treatment and rehabilitation facilities. They discovered that users decide to leave treatment programs when they desire to reduce personally felt risk and increase equity of social capital on a set of values of life. Defection from treatment therefore may not necessarily be thought of as a failure of either abuser or counselor. Recently, Gary Becker, Kevin Murphy, William Landes, Edward Glaeser, and Ivan Werning (2000) elaborated utility maximization and equilibrium. In extending utility functions from economic measures to diverse social phenomena, they analyzed drug use patterns among marriage patterns, prices of collectibles, neighborhood segregation, income and status distribution, the social implications of trademarks, as well as the rise and fall of fashions.

THEORETICAL FRAMEWORK

The rational choice perspective views substance use as a choice made by users. Inherent in the perspective for theoretical exploration are the motive of the subject who makes the choice, the nature of the circumstance in which the choice is made, and the criterion of rationality against which both the choice and the choice maker are evaluated.

Definition

Choice implies options available to as well as the will or discretion commanded by a choice maker. A particular choice is made either because it fulfills the wish of free will or because it stands out as the most cost-effective, the most beneficial, or the most exciting option. Since free will entails nonintellectual desires, passions, and drives, a choice made by a willed individual among his or her various and seemingly viable options may not necessarily be rational—analytically or in terms of essential utilitarian gains. If it is rational, it becomes so only within the subjectivity of the willed individual.

The rational choice perspective builds upon will, choice, and rationality to develop its theoretical explanation of substance, substance use, and substance users. In the course of a free and open quest for insights and understanding, it will delve into such abstract issues as relative rationality, absolute rationality, natural selection, the human organism as a rational entity, and free will. It will also examine concrete interests, from pleasure, performance, public impression, status, personal health, self-care, social participation, and peer pressure, to environmental influence.

Theoretical Image

In the perspective of rational choice, substance, substance use, and substance user become target of choice, choice, or choice maker. Factors that affect choice may emerge from any one of the three choice elements and from the context in which choice is made and carried out.

A substance is a choice target. It is chosen because of its forms, structures, properties, and/or values. At the physiological level, it may act on certain areas of the body, leading to specific effects such as pain relief, sweating, enlarged pupils, or intensified heartbeat. At the psychological level, a substance may generate some usual or unusual feelings and mental states, including euphoria, scare, aloofness, mellowness, or peacefulness. At the social level, a substance may boost performance, heighten alertness, induce courage or endurance, change mood and atmosphere in group gatherings, counteract hazards, and vitalize social interactions. Depending upon the ultimate harm or benefit it presents to the subject of choice, the choice of a substance for consumption can be either rational, nonrational, or rational neutral.

Substance use is an act of choice. A substance is taken in response to bodily needs, psychological tensions, and social pressures. Bodily needs may include hunger, thirst, sex, and other excessive or insufficient conditions caused by defects, deficiencies, malfunctions, and diseases. Psychological tensions may include transpired or translated mental states of bodily needs. They may also include some forceful mind conditions or tendencies, such as craving and withdrawal syndrome. Social pressures invoke efforts and struggles by individuals to stick to tradition, to be part of the crowd, to be different, or to make a statement about self-identity, self-determination, or social attitude. For instance, youths engage in substance use to proclaim that they are tough or evil enough to handle the sin or vice as symbolized by the use of substance. As far as rationality is concerned, substance use in response to bodily needs may not necessarily turn out to be a rational solution of psychological tensions, or necessarily an optimal answer to social pressures.

Substance users are choice makers. They choose between use and nonuse. In use, they choose different substances, licit or illicit, harmful or beneficial, addictive or nonaddictive. Regarding a particular substance, they choose different forms, generic versus name brand, homegrown versus imported, diluted versus concentrated, or inhaled versus swallowed versus injected. As for the reason of choice, human beings are, after all, material beings made up of substances. In order to achieve certain physical, mental, and social states, they have to arm themselves with an appropriate supply of substances. They may eat foods, take medicines, or use drugs. They may appeal to spiritual forces. However, since spiritual forces lie ultimately in material conditions, people who accomplish a task through the spiritual route may just change their biochemical balance, creating future needs for substance supply. Socially, a user's choice of using a substance with no regard to nutritional and medicinal values can be affected by tradition, custom, fashion, law, sentiment, market, knowledge, and circumstance. Rationality can be fashioned in one scenario as "one uses it because everyone else uses it" and in the other as "one uses it because nobody uses it."

Society is where choice of substance and substance use is made. It is where substance users live, interact with one another, and connect to the rest of the population. Society itself also makes choices regarding substance, substance use, and substance users. First, a society knows a definite inventory of substances at any given time. Among those known substances, it may classify them into medicinal versus nonmedicinal, nutritional versus nonnutritional, poisonous versus nonpoisonous, addictive versus nonaddictive, recreational versus nonrecreational, regulated versus nonregulated, or licit versus illicit categories. The classification system, conceptually yet directly, reflects the society's preferences for and rejections of substances. Translated into social action, a society may mobilize its labor force and resources to gather, manufacture, prepare, transport, and trade some substances while hunting, intercepting, confiscating, and destroying others. Second, a society encompasses a wide range of substance use at any point in time. It may sanctify some uses through ceremonies, festivities, rites of passage, gatherings, and recreational activities. It may discourage some uses through shaming, according to moral standards, or by mass media and public opinion. It may prohibit some uses by way of tradition, social convention, and law. Third, a society harbors a variety of substance users at any moment. By giving them different media attentions, legal statuses, and social treatments, it makes some users disciplined, law-abiding, and well-mannered citizens while turning others into unscrupulous, deviant, and out-of-control junkies.

Rationality behind social choice can be examined in terms of knowledge, tradition, custom, sentiment, and social system. A society controls a substance because it knows enough about all the harms associated with the substance. A society widely uses a substance in spite of its known dangers because it has used it for generations. A society allows part of its population to use a substance because it is customary for some of its members to use the substance after a certain age or on certain occasions. A society is engaged in a form of substance use because it is swirled into some temporal yet overwhelming fashions, vogues, or temperaments. By social system, a democratic, free, or open society may embrace a wide range of substance use whereas a traditional, controlled, or closed society may be obsessed with only a few sanctified substances. It is important to note that knowledge, tradition, custom, sentiment, and social system provide different rationalities. Rationality based upon one variable may not necessarily be compatible to that based upon another. For instance, opium smoking or coco chewing may be tradition or custom rational to local habitants in some societies. But from a knowledge point of view, it may be the cause of some chronic ailments, such as respiratory problems and mouth diseases. Across the globe, developed societies have a higher level and a broader range of substance use than developing and undeveloped societies often because the former has a larger knowledge base about substance, a freer attitude toward substance use, and a better-informed and -organized substance user population.

In history, the repertoire of substances known to human beings expands gradually and steadily. In the beginning, people have access only to those few substances that exist in their direct environment and are often closely associated with their foods and medicines. Choices are limited. The choice of one or two substances for spiritual, ceremonial, or entertainment use is sanctified. With advancement in trade, science, and manufacturing, people in the contemporary era know far more substances than their ancestors did. Available for their choosing, there are naturally grown versus laboratory- or factory-synthesized substances, domestic versus imported substances, mild versus hard substances, prescribed versus over-the-counter substances, and controlled versus noncontrolled substances. Use is diverse and innovative. Beyond practical purpose, such as pain relief and recovery from illness, there are uses for stimulation, depression, daydreaming, hallucination, illusion, transcendence, or just recreation. Users, while being unrestrained by tradition, unrestricted by custom, and unconcerned with bodily needs, are constantly pushed by peer pressure, social fashion, commonsense knowledge, material affluence, and individualistic independence to experiment with one substance after another or to take a combination of substances in their use career.

The base of choice has changed over time. In the past, choice was made in accordance with tradition and convention. Instead of being grounded in solid information and knowledge, choice was often shrouded in unsubstantiated speculation and superstition. In contemporary society, although they do not abide by tradition and convention, people follow their peers, neighbors, colleagues, and fellow citizens, through the mass media, in social trends and vogues. They are confident because they feel they are educated, informed, and equipped with knowledge and technology. They are determined because they feel they are cared for, supported, and protected by advanced medicine and material affluence. From a purely analytical point of view, rationality becomes more apparent, more real, and more robust when it shifts base from entrenched tradition to sentimentalized social fashion, from superstition to science, from speculation to knowledge, from social conformity to individualistic determination, and from limited choices to multiple selections. Ironically, however, it is exactly the variety of available substances, the multiplicity of publicized substance uses, and the diversity of informed, unrestrained, and determined substance users that make the contemporary era a truly dangerous time for substance use and abuse.

Theoretical Components

The rational choice perspective examines the whole choosing process of substance use by users. Falling under its theoretical jurisdiction are major variables pertaining to choice, choice-making situation, choice maker, and choice criterion.

The Human Body as a Selective Entity

Regarding the subject of choice, the human body is a peculiar biochemical system. The system is governed by a set of laws in physics, chemistry, biology, and physiology. As far as substance intake is concerned, the human body first does not take everything. It rejects a lot of objects in existence and takes only a limited number of substances as nutrients, medicines, or other active agents. Second, it takes substances in specific routes, swallowing, inhaling, skin absorbing, or through the bloodstream. Third, it adjusts to a substance it takes into its system. By adjustment, the human body may develop tolerance or special biochemical conditions. Fourth, as soon as an adjustment condition is established in the presence of a substance, the human body reacts in the form of a withdrawal syndrome when the substance is absent. Finally, objective body conditions underpin subjective mind motions. The mind changes sequentially as the body moves coherently from one equilibrium to another.

The fact that the human body follows the law of nature not only makes it a selective entity, but also turns it into an ultimate base for rationality. In other words, because the human body itself is a selective organism operating on the principle of rationality, it provides the last, if not the only, explanation for why a substance is taken, why tolerance is developed, why addiction is followed, and why relapse is fueled by a withdrawal syndrome. From a scientifically deterministic point of view, one may even legitimately claim that human rationality in substance choice and other social affairs boils down to the human body, a rationally built and operating system governed by the law of nature. Subjective feelings are phenomenal. They offer only an explanation of superficial rationality: one takes a substance because he or she feels exhilarated after intake. Objective bodily conditions are essential. They provide an explanation of ultimate rationality: one takes a substance because the substance acts on the part of the brain that controls his or her state of mood or emotionality.

Free Will

Free will has long been mystified as innate drives, inner urges, natural wants, instinctual desires, and unstoppable life energy. It is free because it emits from the origin of life and represents the vigor of life. It is a will because it is a fierce force to overcome obstacles, to conquer enemies, to acquire power and wealth, and to take charge. Now the question is: if indeed there is such an underlying force as free will in life, how would it play out in reality, under various social constraints faced by individuals who live their life on a daily basis?

On the matter of substance and substance use, how would free will translate into choice? Choice of use can be perceived as a demonstration of will, in response to innate needs or some deeply felt wants, free from social inhibitions or knowledge-based health alerts. Choice of nonuse can be viewed as a show of will as well, out of ego ideals or some personally adopted philosophy, free from bodily dispositions and psychological allures. Among those who choose to use substances continually, some may boast about their free will in the form of accommodation, adaptation, tolerance, endurance, perseverance, or other characteristics if they survive the longest use, largest combination of drugs, highest dosage of a drug, most potent form of a drug, or most harmful substance. Among those who choose between use and nonuse, some may toast their free will as having a most open, elastic, or flexible biopsycho system because they feel free to use and stop any substance anytime, without falling into the trap of chemical or psychological dependency.

Another question concerning free will is: what is the purpose of free will? The classic school of thought assumes that free will is geared to bring about pleasure to the self. The commonsense perception seems to follow suit. But what is pleasure? Is it temporal or eternal? Is it situational or holistic? Is it spiritual or materialistic? Is it bodily, psychological, social, or combinational of all? Substance and substance use obviously traverse the whole terrain of pleasure and its opposite. Some substances generate mellowness, comfort, peace, euphoria, and pleasure while others create feelings of anxiety, distress, restlessness, and pain. Temporal, situational pleasure brought about by substance use may cause a long-lasting, systematic strain on one's biochemical system. Since drugs are expensive, spiritual transcendence promised by a substance may well cost one a material fortune. Because drugs are regulated, bodily comfort and psychological euphoria achieved by the use of a substance may soon be outdone by intense social shaming and distancing. In the classical and common-sensical sense, free will is used to refer to an original yet ubiquitous force, and pleasure is meant to designate a simple yet universal state. But when applied to a real-world issue, such as substance use, free will seems to encompass all, including socially tempered motivation and ambition. Similarly, pleasure appears to embrace all, from economically seasoned self-interest to culturally brewed self-actualization.

Rationality and Criterion

A fundamental principle that is assumed to guide the making and the assessment of choice is rationality. Taken for granted, people who claim to be rational beings seem to know what it means to be rational. Being rational first requires that one draw upon his or her intelligence and intellectuality, rather than emotion and instinct, in his or her approach to various issues in life. Second, it implies that one make choices and decisions in accordance with his or her circumstance. Third, it dictates that one act in a way that serves his or her ultimate interest in terms of personal health, social advancement, and overall well-being. Specifically, rationality invokes such acts as planning, prioritizing, following logic, being methodical, calculating cost and benefit, weighing means and ends, relying upon facts, and being instrumental.

From the general image of rationality, it is natural to infer about its absolute existence. Absolute rationality refers to the universality of rationality in human affairs: every human act, every human thought, and every human event can be evaluated in various degrees of rationality. It also attends to the essential interest of human life as the ultimate base for rationality. Regarding substance use, what rationality is there? First, as a human act, substance use always involves a rationality judgment, either from the perspective of the subject or from the situational and contextual points of view. For instance, one uses a substance in rational relation to his or her medical conditions or to some prodrug sentiments in his or her neighborhood. Second, if substance use does not promote health or make one live longer and in greater happiness, how would it be judged in absolute rationality? What utilitarian or utility-comparable base can be referred to in rationality determination? Is substance use totally irrational or is it rational in the sense that it challenges life; it tests life; it enriches life; it makes life colorful; it demonstrates the risk, fragility, and liability of life; or it reinforces a conventional approach to life through unconventional experimentation?

Relative rationality, on the other hand, centers on the particularity of rationality in the human sphere: an act, a thought, or an event is rational only to specific references under specific contexts in specific time. It also argues that nothing essential can be identified as the ultimate base for rationality. The criteria by which rationality is determined change from place to place and from time to time. As far as substance and substance use are concerned, relative rationality can be explored on different fronts. First, rationality can be body-based or mind-based. The former may not necessarily be compatible to the latter. For instance, a substance may make one feel as if he or she enters a state of peace and tranquility, whereas a physician may warn that it severely disturbs the normal function of part of one's body or it viciously changes one's biochemical balance. Similarly, a substance, prescribed by a physician, may correct a bodily condition as measured by laboratory tests, while it makes one feel painful, nauseous, or paranoid. Second, rationality can be analyzed in short versus long terms, material versus nonmaterial dimensions, and logical versus situational factors. For instance, one takes a painkiller knowing its long-term side effects or one braves the bitterness of a substance in the expectation of its long-term benefits. One focuses on the enhancement or alteration effect of a substance without regard for its purity, quality, and other material conditions. An extreme scenario is that a homeless person picks up an unfinished cigarette butt from the street or empties unfinished beer from a thrown-away bottle just to obtain a taste or shock of tobacco or alcohol. Or one pays too much attention to the color, shape, package, and material outlooks of a substance but does not really care or know if the substance indeed gives him or her a feeling of relief, happiness, or transcendence. A typical case is that one uses a substance because it looks cool, smells funny, or feels different. In relevance to circumstance, one may take a substance to prove his or her courage or brotherhood or sisterhood no matter how much it costs his or her paycheck or health. In adherence to logic, one may be so calculative about expense, so meticulous about schedule, or so serious about self-feeling that he or she ignores situational restraints to administer his or her own preparations of a substance at any time.

Finally, rationality can be anchored to different bases: goal, tradition, value, or affection. Focusing on goal, a substance user may take a substance because it relieves pain, enhances performance, or corrects an unfavorable mental or physical condition. His or her choice can then be viewed as instrumental-rational. Sticking to tradition, one may take a substance because he or she inherits pipes, drinkware, and secret preparation methods from his or her parents, aunts, uncles, grandparents, or even earlier ancestors. In the sense that he or she carries on an important family, kinship, or tribal tradition, he or she makes a tradition-rational choice in substance use. A value-rational decision regarding substance use centers on norms, beliefs, values, or ideologies. For instance, one chooses not to use substances because he or she believes substance is sin and substance use is vice. Or one uses a substance just to make a statement about his or her suspicion, resistance, or rebellion toward authority, government, or mass media. Finally, some may use a substance due to a particular instinctual urge, carnal want, or emotional uproar. Although it may first sound out of reason, the use can still be logical and rational in terms of instinct and affection. For instance, one may well legitimately say: "I use the substance in that occasion at that moment because it makes me feel cool and fun." The choice of use can therefore be judged as an affection-rational one.

Social Influence

Individuals live in culture and society. They make choice under social and cultural constraints. In most cases, they subject their choices to social rather than personal standards for rationality judgment. They are likely to feel, sooner or later, that they are unwise and irrational if they stubbornly pursue their free-will-based interests without regard to social norms and restraints.

Social influences figure in the individual choice of substance and substance use from different sources, in different forms, and with different intensities. As far as source is concerned, social influence may come from tradition, custom, law, peer, or fashion. Tradition can be long established in a community or culture. It can also be observed from time to time by a family, group, or organization. For instance, as drinking is established as a tradition in holiday celebrations, for people in many circumstances, to drink is to respect tradition and to join in festivities. Custom dictates behavior in routine activities or reaction to important events. For instance, when it is customary to serve tea to guests or to drink beer after the harvest or final examinations, it becomes a natural choice for guests, farmers, or college students to take tea, to gormandize foods and alcohol, or to go on binge drinking. Law classifies substances and regulates substance use. People use more licit than illicit substances partly because the latter are controlled. People use prescription drugs only when they are ordered and supervised by licensed physicians. People use over-the-counter drugs more freely and confidently because they can obtain understandable information about and gain nonscrutinized access to those drugs. Peer exerts its influence with resort to similarity in age, race, job, or social status. People in a similar category tend to follow each other in their behavior and idiosyncrasy. Adolescents are known to experiment with drugs due to peer pressure. Celebrities are famed to sip fine wines and smoke brand cigars in their upscale lifestyles. Professional colleagues follow one another by having a coffee break during work, chatting in smoking areas, or visiting a bar on the way home. Finally, fashion, as a generalized social behavior, may sweep a segment of society or the whole population into a short-lived yet intensified interest in a newfound substance. For instance, when a new drug makes its debut in a fashionable way, as it often does, adolescents, young adults, and club enthusiasts are likely to join in the fun and adventure one crowd after another. Individuals would quickly feel left out if they chose to hold back from the fashion.

Regarding form, social influence may make its impact through the general environment or a specific situation. Individuals live in a general social environment. They listen to the radio, watch television, read newspapers and magazines, attend political rallies, go to supermarkets, walk in the street, conduct business, and run other chores in their daily routine. They act under the law, deal with the government, and feel the sentiment of society. Voluntarily or involuntarily, they may choose to use or not to use a substance or a group of substances in response to overall ideological, political, economic, and legal climates and atmospheres in their organization, community, and society. The specific situation includes various social settings where a group of people gather for sports, recreation, and other activities. Surrounded by people of similar interests or characteristics, one can be easily led to engage in acts that may stretch beyond his or her natural capacities. Drinking and using drugs, unfortunately, are often typical examples of those out-of-control acts. Related to the source of influence, impacts from tradition, custom, law, and fashion are likely to be environmental, whereas those from peers are likely to be situational. However, peer influence can be environmental as well. For instance, one can legitimately argue that people take their peers seriously in each social occasion because they generally are other-directed in the contemporary era. Likewise, tradition, custom, law, and fashion can exert their respective influence in specific situations, too. For instance, tradition is often passed on in family settings. Custom is usually exercised through concretely arranged rites of passage by particular age cohorts or ethnic groups.

The intensity of social influence may range from strong, through moderate, to weak. Depending upon the source, the form, and their various combinations, the same social influence can exhibit different intensities. For instance, tradition is generally remote and weak in its influence in contemporary society where focus is put on the present and future. Influence can be moderate if a tradition is recently established. It can be intense and strong at the time when and in the occasion where tradition is honored and emphasized. In general, influences from custom and tradition are gradual, voluntary, moderate, or weak, whereas those from law, fashion, and peer are immediate, involuntary, and strong, or at least moderate.

Environmental influence tends to be distant, suggestive, and casual while situational influence is likely to be close, coercive, and intense.

Rationality under Addiction

Choice of substance and substance use, in most cases, is made by users who are under and therefore are already affected by the condition of use. There are novice, casual, and habitual users. There are habituation, addiction, and dependency as states of use. If rationality is body-based, is there any rationality at all or does rationality shift to a lower or higher level when the subject uses a substance and floats on a biochemical balance other than the normal equilibrium averaged by all nonusers? If rationality is mind-based, does rationality still exist or does it move to a different state when the subject is obsessed with the stimulating or depressing effect of the substance? Most essentially, is rationality a changing condition or is it dictated by some universal state or principle, such as pleasure, peace, and self-interest?

Suppose rationality is a changing condition. There is no ideal state, nor end, nor standard. One begins as a rational-choice maker. He chooses to use substance out of his free will and in response to social influences from his environment. As a rational user, he progresses from initiation, to experimentation, and to habituation. In the stage of habituation, he lives on certain doses a day. In one scenario where substance is in steady supply, he takes in the quantity he needs and in the quality he desires. He then may stay permanently in a use-based rational state: he functions as a member of society while enjoying his substance of choice. He then may also proceed to addictive or even destructive use. In a somewhat rational response, he uses more and more substance because he feels he needs to use more and more just to continue his life. At some point, however, he falls into total sickness or demise as the body is no longer able to handle the intake. Rationality may thereby be exhausted to naught. In self-consciousness as well as by scientific measure, however, the road toward death or the fall of rationality through addiction may not only be subjectively felt as necessary, consistent, and natural, but also objectively analyzed as logical, coherent, and rational. In other words, while users feel they proceed rationally in each step of use intensification or deterioration, scientists may explain, on the basis of laboratory tests, one's unstoppable tendency to take more of a substance as an inevitable response to the changing biochemical condition created by the substance.

In another scenario where substance is controlled, one as a habitual user has to obtain his needed substance in compromised quality and quantity. Rational to his circumstance, he may take whatever quality of a substance in whatever amount he can obtain at his disposal. In a desperate need to fix an overwhelming craving or a devastating withdrawal reaction, one may inject a trace of blood-tainted liquid in a syringe used by somebody else. The choice may be perceived rational in the sense that the user feels he is saving his life, although at the risk of his health. It may be viewed rational in the sense that the situation is understandable to any observer witnessing the suffering of the user. On the matter of financing, he may offer his belongings in exchange for drugs. He may pawn his children, spouse, and relatives on drug debts. He may sell his body in the sex market. He may engage in criminal activities, such as stealing, robbery, embezzlement, distortion, or drug dealing. Within each choice of making money for drugs, one may feel he has used the best of his intelligence, reasoning, resource, and circumstance: "I have a drug habit; keeping my habit is my highest priority and keeping my habit represents my ultimate interest; I have exhausted all other avenues in thinking and actual trial; and the only choice now is to . . ." To a social scientist who follows the user and examines the whole of his situation, the choice may also be sensible, plausible, and understandable in light of logic and scientific reasoning.

Finally, suppose that rationality is guided and determined by some general principles or standards, and that it is exemplified in a universal state or ultimate ideal. Substance use can then be outrightly judged as irrational if it is generally agreed that the ultimate goals of life and the essential interests of human beings are health, happiness, and longevity and if it is definitely determined that substance use does not enhance or serve either of those fundamental life goals or human interests. Affectually understandable and scientifically explicable choices by users under the influence of substance are just outcomes of clouded, twisted, or otherwise compromised rationality. Rationality loses, although the process of loss may follow some logically analyzable sequences, as subjects choose to use drugs, use more and more drugs in the addictive state, act out of their needs or desires but against their ultimate interests, and gradually give in their consciousness, intelligence, and free will to the power of substance. Rationality vanishes when addiction takes users to total dysfunction and final demise.

Theoretical Applications

The rational choice perspective establishes a unique frame of reference to explore both abstract and concrete issues concerning substance, substance use, and substance users.

At the abstract level, substance is part of nature. Is it offered by nature as a gift or a vice? Does it serve as a messenger, warning, or agent of selection? If it is an agent of selection, what human qualities are to be developed and reinforced by nature through its offering of a particular substance? From the human point of view, substance is discovered, made, modified, or purified from nature. Does it symbolize human creativity and pride? Does it test human will and wisdom in making appropriate selections among various offerings by nature? If a chosen substance does not necessarily serve human beings in their best interest, how far and how much does it reflect human vulnerability, corruptibility, or culpability? Second, substance use is a human act. To what extent does it demonstrate the determination of free will? To what degree does it exhibit the power of social influences and situational forces? On the part of free will, is substance use purely a human choice? Does it, at least indirectly through the natural accommodation and adaptation of the human body, represent the selection of nature? On the part of social influence, is substance use exclusively an individual decision? Is it just a social act carried out by the mass of individuals? Finally, substance users are living agents. Are they ultimate choice makers? Are they puppets of either natural selection or social preference? If they live to illustrate the mighty power of nature, are they merely objects controlled by the genetic code to grow, to be addictive to certain substances, and to die? If they exist to show the influence of culture and society, are they subjects acting collectively to create and maintain social fashions and historical patterns, including trends and vogues in substance use and abuse?

In the concrete sense, a substance is an object to be viewed, touched, smelled, tasted, and felt. What appeal does it have in appearance? Is it colorful? Is it attractive in shape? Does its smell or taste present an irresistible stimulation to the body? Does it generate a feeling of aloofness, a dream, or an illusion? Does it help one manage pain, cope with stress, or enhance performance? For the purpose of choice, is it possible to assess and compare the relative importance of each aspect of a substance, from its physical features, price, availability, forms of use, convenience of use, physiological reactions, and psychological effects, to social significance? Regarding substance use, does it look cool, mature, or elegant? Does it take serious effort? Does its benefit outweigh its harm? Does it convey any message about attitude and ideology? Does it signify loyalty, conformity, bravery, wealth, status, or some other quality? For instance, when substance use is controlled, it may be occasionally attempted by those excluded from use as a conspicuous act to demonstrate courage and an adventurous spirit. With respect to users, are they loners or collective actors? Do they follow their own mind or the consciousness of their immediate group? What traditional, customary, and current forces are they subject to in substance choice? What work and life situations are they involved in? More specifically, what personal characteristics do they have? Are they predisposed to substance use? Do they live in a family, a kinship, a group, or a neighborhood where substance use is taken for granted? Do they network with peers who use illicit substances? What pro- and anti-substance-use factors do they receive from their environment?

Empirical Tests

The rational choice perspective creates opportunities for empirical research. Various choice aspects of substance use can be studied through both established and newfound research methods.

Case studies can follow individual substances, substance uses, users, groups, and societies for close-up scrutinies. Why is one substance more likely to be chosen than another? Is it because of price, availability, physical feature, chemical property, psychological effect, addictive power, legal status, or public perception? Why is one form of a substance more favored than the other? How does one substance emerge as the drug of choice for most young users or the whole user population? Focusing on substance use, research can be done on routes of administration, forms of use, occasions of use, and other use-related characteristics. For instance, what features do inhaling, snorting, injecting, swallowing, or other routes of administration have? How is chewing compared to smoking and other forms of tobacco use? Is binge drinking more likely to happen on the college campus than in other settings? Centering on users, case studies can follow private stories to learn in detail about every choice in the journey toward addiction or recovery. Fall into substance use may be due to an accident, an encounter with a stranger, or a temporary loss of mind, aside from tradition, custom, and peer-related choice factors. Dependent substance use may not necessarily be a matter of choice but a no-way-out situation. Recovery may take will but determination can often be prompted and sustained by situational factors. With regard to groups and societies, they may choose to adopt some substances as their collective drugs of choice. They may also have to make systemwide decisions regarding drug control and substance regulation. One thing for sure is: only through case studies can all these unique varieties be documented and appreciated in academic literature.

Historical analysis brings a long-term perspective to the matter of choice. Regarding users, do they change in making and pursuing substance use choice over their life course? Are they more sensitive to some factors when they are young? Do they care more about other factors when they enter their senior ages? As far as their will is concerned, are they more narrow-minded and stubborn when they are either very young or very old? Are they more flexible yet stable in substance use when they move with adequate knowledge and experience through adulthood? Beyond individual users, groups, organizations, communities, and societies may change over time in their attitudes and behaviors toward substance use. There might be periods of pro–substance use when sanctions against substance use and abuse are loosened. There might be periods of anti–substance use when citizens are shamed or punished for even therapeutic or recreational use. Throughout history, some general use patterns can thus be identified in relation to law, morality, sentiments, and other collective dynamics.

Survey research is useful to establish commonalities in substance use choice. By asking questions among a sizable sample, one or two salient factors can be identified as to why a substance is a hotly pursued item in youth party scenes, why a substance maintains its popularity over time or across age groups, why one use is favored over the other, or why use is chosen along with other follow-up acts, such as car racing, sex, dancing, and talking. Users can reveal, in general terms, which is more important in their choice of substance use or nonuse, self-control or environmental factors. On the question of self-control, they may differentiate between free will and socialization, strong ego and maturation, or personality and perception by others. Among environmental factors, they may single out family, community, peer, media, or situational force as primary influences in their initiation into, habituation of, or recovery from substance abuse. Users may also share information on particular issues, such as common effects of a substance, irrational aspects of a law, and misleading reports by the media. For instance, users may blame harsh drug control on their choice of unclean needles and syringes in shooting galleries.

Experimental studies can shed light on the relative importance of one factor over another in substance and substance use choice. At the system level, two otherwise similar periods can be compared to see if the introduction of a legislative measure or social policy or the breakout of a public movement or event in one period makes any difference on substance use choice. Two otherwise similar societies can also be compared to learn if one or two factors, present in one society while absent in the other, influence people in their choice of substance and substance use. At the microlevel, groups of users can be randomly selected and assigned to different experimental conditions to examine if and how each situational as well as nonsituational factor figures in the process of substance choice. Users may also be compared to nonusers, addictive users to nonaddictive users, recovered users to relapsed users, or criminal users to noncriminal users to ascertain if rationality or frame of mind changes from circumstance to circumstance.

POLICY IMPLICATIONS

People choose to use or not to use substances. Society chooses to deal with or not to deal with substance use. The rational choice perspective can obviously provide both sides with insights for their respective choices.

Public Health

On the treatment side, medical professionals are geared to correct disorder and to bring the abnormal back to the normal. The abnormal condition they are faced with is often transitional, meaning that it can either be reversed to its origin through intervention, or be allowed to reach a new state of equilibrium by its own force. However, since the second option is customarily viewed as an irresponsible reaction by medical professionals themselves, few of them would choose to simply stand by to watch a situation spiral out of their own comprehension or control. To demonstrate their training, competency, professional instincts and ethics, or humanistic spirit of care, medical professionals would choose to do something, no matter if they know exactly what that something would do to patients and their transitionally abnormal conditions. From an objective point of view, intervention may indeed correct an abnormal condition, pushing it back to normal. It may contain a situation, preventing it from developing into a more serious condition. There is also the possibility that it might exacerbate a condition, holding it back from normal while keeping it from reaching a new state of balance. The last possibility may be particularly relevant to substance use: substance users choose to use substances; the biochemical system of users chooses to accommodate and adapt to the substances; and if a transitionally adjusting or disturbing condition is left alone to develop by its own logic, it may eventually reach its own balance, self-sufficiency, or functionality.

On the prevention side, health educators, social workers, therapists, and counselors tend to assume that they know more than their substance use clients about bodily needs, psychological desires, health attitudes, and social demands. They question clients and their abilities to make rational choices about their own mental and physical welfare. They may even treat their clients as objects that do not have any intelligence, as children who have only limited reasoning capacities, or as totally ignorant and irrational humans who just need help. As a result, they automatically impose their frame of mind and their perspective of rationality upon their clients, and they lose sight of other versions of normality, functionality, and rationality. An essential learning from the rational choice perspective is: substance users are rational choice makers, just like anyone else; they make substance use choices on the basis of their knowledge, experience, needs, desires, and circumstances; to influence users in their substance use choice-making behavior, prevention workers first need to assume, rather than ignore or negate, their clients' frame of mind or perspective of rationality; and only when they know which one is more important than another in their clients' world of rationality can prevention workers pointedly introduce needed variables to change their clients' substance use choice. The key is: prevention workers cannot make decisions for their clients; it is the clients who make decisions that may ultimately change their life.

Social Control

Learning from the rational choice perspective can be either nonreflective or reflective for social control. A nonreflective approach is to assume that substance users are rational choice makers who respond to social control messages and measures. To control substance use is therefore to create a general social environment in which substance is portrayed as irrelevant to basic human needs, substance use is viewed as harmful, and substance users are distanced as outsiders. Specifically, substances are classified into groups. Licit substances are levied heavy taxes. Illicit substances are outrightly forced out of the open market into underground operations. Price is pushed high. Quality is made uncertain. Availability is controlled so that most people would not dump a considerable portion of their earnings on licit substances or even risk their whole life on illicit substances. Substance use is monitored and restricted to certain time and places. While licit substance use may occur in private homes or capitalize on public occasions, illicit substance use is pushed only to attics, toilets, street corners, and other isolated areas. Substance users are shamed, distanced, and punished. Marriage discriminates against drunkards and smokers. Employment shuns drug dependents and addicts. Law targets drug dealers and abusers. Media deride and attack substance users and their subculture. In the age of drug war, substance users are even chased down to their bedroom by the mighty governmental machinery, including its ideological and military components, as real enemies in the battlefield.

A reflective response from social control is to examine its whole operation to see if it is rational to keep the war on drugs. First, substance use is a problem. It needs and deserves certain public attention and some social actions. But the questions are: is it necessary to stage a war on substance use and abuse? Is it necessary to create and expand multigovernmental agencies to fight, regulate, and treat substance use? Is it necessary to mobilize law enforcement, business, mass media, and community to deal with substance use? Is it cost-effective to spend millions of dollars a year on drug abuse research and treatment? Is it necessary to equalize drug interdiction and substitution to diplomatic relations with some foreign countries? Is it necessary to parallel drug campaigns to national interests? It is urgent that social control in substance use and abuse be evaluated and readjusted so that it is carried out with tangible outcomes. Most important, substance use is not blown out of proportion. It is dealt with as it is in proper social contexts, not in a way that obscures critical social problems and exhausts limited social resources. Second, social control agents should readjust their view and treatment of substance users not only as rational

choice makers who respond to social control measures, but also as rational choice makers who approach their own substance use habits with care
and caution. Imagine that substance use were not controlled. Substance
users would obtain their drugs of choice without fear and under normal
market conditions. Although a few might fall off the cliff into death or total
dysfunction by naturally following their substance use habit, the whole
result from noncontrol might still be far better than that from control. The
key to a noncontrol choice is a genuine belief in human rationality and
an unwavering trust in substance users as fellow human beings.

Life and Community

Most variables pertaining to substance use choice center around life in
the community. People use substances in following or rebelling against
tradition, custom, or fashion inherent in their communal lifestyle. People
emulate parents, siblings, cousins, peers, or neighbors in substance initiation, experimentation, and habituation. In a sense, it is legitimate to say
that life is the ultimate source of rationality or irrationality in substance
use choice. Suppose substance users are rational. They make an irrational choice of substance use because they are subject to irrational conditions supplied from life in their community. Suppose substance users are
irrational. They are irrational because they are nurtured to be irrational
by the very conditions inherent in their life. They make an irrational choice
of substance use because they cannot make any sensible decision about
their own welfare in a community of irrational existence. To effect change
in substance use and substance users, community and people in the community must first look into themselves to see what can be done about
larger environmental and situational conditions.

Another learning from the rational perspective is that substance users
should be trusted to finish the whole journey of their rational or irrational choice. While variables leading to substance use originate from life,
forces condemning, shaming, and punishing substance use often first
emerge and intensify in communal settings. Parents curse their substance
use children as susceptible, rebellious, uneducable, or otherwise hopeless
before they drop out of school and run away from home. Spouses shame
their substance use partner as weak-willed, incompetent, annoying, or
totally helpless before they take refuge in a homeless shelter or retreat fully
away from productive life. Ironically to many substance users, they can
endure the harshest treatment from a secondary social control agency but
cannot put up with one single alienating word from a significant other in
their primary relations. It is therefore important that people in the life of
substance users withhold their sentimental reactions, forgo moral judgment, and lend their parental, spousal, familial, or other type of love and
support unwaveringly and unconditionally. Without emotional and moral

disturbances, substance users may be able to follow their own version of rationality, clouded or unclouded under the influence of substance, to stay in control of their substance use habit or to walk out of a drug dependency situation. Externally forced actions may change something overnight. But only self-reasoned decisions endure long in their consequences.

Work and Organization

Central to the task of an organization, it might sound outrightly rational for it to ban a substance and its use on the premises if it is legally controlled, to terminate an employee from its payroll if he or she fails to perform his or her duty under the influence of a substance, or to remain neutral if substance use does not affect its employee morale and productivity or bring it into contact with the law.

But in the sense that work is a human act and organization is a unit of society, work, organization, and choices made by or on behalf of them cannot be evaluated just in terms of variables within themselves. Instead, they must be judged by an array of factors both within and without. For instance, one uses a substance due to the stress of work, negative influences from co-workers, or the discriminating environment of his or her organization. He or she then is fired by the organization because his or her substance use violates the law, breaks the regulations of the organization, affects his or her job performance, or simply creates an unfavorable condition in the context of work. What is the justice in the rational choice by the organization? Suppose the fired employee is the only bread earner in his or her household. Loss of employment then may not only turn his or her life upside down, but also push a whole family into despair. Children may be forced out of school. The spouse may be cornered into desperate endeavors, including prostituting, cheating, begging, or stealing, to maintain the life of the family. A simple rational choice in the perspective of the organization may thus lead to a very irrational consequence on the part of family and society.

On the other hand, if an organization renders its support to an employee in trouble with substance, it may not just sacrifice its economic interests. Instead, it may create various benefits on many fronts. To the employee in need of help, the organization presents a precious gift to keep his or her courage in making rational choices pertaining to his or her substance use. The employee may choose nonuse or controlled use to keep not only himself but also his organization trouble-free from the matter. To the whole employee population, the organization shows its caring and humanistic side. Employee dedication, loyalty, and morale can be subtly boosted. To the community, the organization demonstrates its invaluable role in contributing to substance prevention and treatment. To the society, it fulfills a serious responsibility of taking care of a group of people and their families. Economic interests, if there are any lost through an employee substance assistance program, can hence be doubly, trebly, or even multiply harvested in various other forms of benefits.

In sum, the rational choice perspective opens up a peculiar window to look at substance, substance use, and substance users. Substance is chosen for use or control due to its effects on the human mind and body. Substance use is adopted, sanctified, regulated, or prohibited because of its pharmacological, recreational, sentimental, religious, or cultural significance. Substance users make substance and substance use choices on the basis of their personal needs as well as their social conventions. In a larger context, the society or historical period chooses substance, substance use, and substance users for control or protection, reward or punishment, and shaming or glorifying in response to specific internal and external conditions, especially its relations with nature.

Choice is made by a subject. The subject possesses will, weighs options, and follows rules. In classical literature, free will, the pleasure principle, and rationality are thought of as guidelines in the choice-making process. In contemporary research, reasoning, cost-effect contrasts, means-ends comparisons, and situational factors are considered as independent variables affecting choice decisions. There might be an existence of absolute rationality. But realistically, being rational or irrational can be evaluated only on specific choices in particular times and places. For substance users, they may feel they have made a rational choice of substance and substance use but soon find they have to make numerous irrational efforts to keep or quit their use habit. Similarly, they may regret they have made an irrational choice of substance and substance use but in actuality feel they struggle conscientiously and rationally to live up to their life expectations under the influence of substance. Another example of relative rationality is entrenchment: users are programmed into use. They think and reason in the perspective of use. Under the rationality of use, they are more likely to think what they do for use is rational, and therefore, are less likely to make a rational choice of nonuse. That may conceptually explain why quitting substance use is so difficult or why relapsing is so commonplace among substance use treatment clients.

From a reflective point of view, the rational choice perspective alerts public health, social control, community, organization, and other agents or agencies to frame their approach to substance use in the principle of rationality and choice. Is it rational just to prevent, treat, control, shame, and punish substance use and substance users? Are there alternatives? The most important point is: substance users are ultimate choice makers. Only when they are understood and respected in their right to choice can they be gradually persuaded and led to a path toward self-control and self-welfare. Intervention is then not to set agendas, impose rules, or apply coercive forces, but to introduce new variables, create new situations, raise new hopes, and make new choices. A choice will stand and bear fruit when the choice maker feels he or she is in charge of making it and following through with it.

—6—

The Social Control Perspective

Unlike food intake, substance use is not necessitated by life. It has no definite benefit for human survival. Instead, it causes disruption and disturbance to the body and its natural processes. Even in recreational use when the mind is allegedly entertained or social role-playing activities are purposely facilitated, substance consumed means not only resources spent, but also wastes to be cleaned. For instance, in a social gathering where certain amounts of alcohol and tobacco are consumed, someone has to pay for the purchase of alcoholic beverages and tobacco products. Each user, especially casual users, may need several days to circulate the substance out of his or her system.

The social control perspective begins with the unnecessary and harmful nature of substance use. It assumes that substance use is an unnatural, irrational, abnormal, and deviant behavior. People normally do not use substance. A few who use substance begin with a loosening or a lack of proper restraints in family, school, work, or other social settings. Once they use substance, they may experience a further loss of control in their life. To prevent substance use is to institute and strengthen proper social control measures. To intervene in substance abuse is to restore order and to gain control.

SOURCES OF INSPIRATION

The idea of social control appears as early as the time of Aristotle when scholars begin to reflect upon the nature of human social life (Roucek 1978). In sociology, Auguste Comte, Emile Durkheim, Karl Marx, Max Weber, and other founding figures generate a wealth of thoughts on social control as they study authority, power, order, and influence in society. However, as a formal sociological concept, social control is first proposed and elaborated by Edward Ross (1901). According to Ross, belief systems, as influenced by and reflected in law, public opinion, education, religion, custom, ceremony, art, enlightenment, illusion, and morality, guide what people do and universally serve to control behavior.

After Ross, social control takes on a variety of meanings and interpretations in the sociological literature (Janowitz 1975). Macrosociological perspectives focus on formal systems, including laws, the criminal justice system, the government, and powerful social groups. They study how formal control agents and measures inhibit rule-breaking behavior in society as well as foster oppression, fear, and alienation across the general population (Davis and Anderson 1983; Cohen and Scull 1983). Microsociological perspectives, on the other hand, concentrate on informal systems, such as self-esteem, family, school, and peer groups. They examine individual socialization processes in an attempt to explain why people conform by internalizing the external source of control.

Beginning with individuals, Albert Reiss (1951) is one of the first sociologists to study the relationship between personal and social controls. He argues that juvenile delinquency results from (a) a lack of social rules that prescribe behavior in the family, the school, and other important social groups; (b) a failure to internalize socially prescribed norms of behavior; and (c) a breakdown of internal controls. Toby (1957) observes that only a few among many youths in socially disorganized neighborhoods commit crimes. He attributes the difference between one particular individual who becomes a delinquent and another who does not to the individual's own stake in conformity, or correspondence of behavior to society's patterns, norms, or standards. Walter Reckless (1962) presents an even broader analysis of how personal factors interact with social control in his containment theory. According to Reckless, for every individual there exists a containing external structure and a protective internal structure, both of which provide defense, protection, and insulation against deviant behavior. Included in the external structure, or outer containment, are a social role that guides daily activities, a set of reasonable limits and responsibilities, an opportunity for status attainment, participation in joint activities with a group, a sense of belonging, identification with particular people in a group, and alternative ways of satisfaction. Inherent in the internal structure, or inner containment, are a positive self-concept, self-control, a strong ego, a well-developed conscience, a high frustration tolerance, and a clear sense of responsibility. Deviance occurs when inner containment fails to control internal pushes, such as a need for immediate gratification, restlessness, and hostility; when outer containment fails to deal with external pulls, such as poverty, unemployment, and blocked opportunities; or most likely when both internal and external controls remain ineffective in addressing pressures from within and without.

David Matza (1964) assumes that adolescents normally sense a moral obligation to abide by the conventional "bind" between a person and the law. Most of the time they follow rules, observe the order, and remain duty-bound to social responsibility. They drift into delinquency not because of an involuntary failure of their inner and/or outer containment, but rather because of a voluntary development of defense mechanisms that release them from the constraints of convention. For example, they use denial of responsibility, denial of injury, denial of the victim, condemnation of the condemner, and appeal to higher loyalties as defenses to neutralize their inner sense of guilt, to ward off possible social attacks, and to rationalize particular delinquent acts (Sykes and Matza 1957).

A shift of focus is made from individual motivations to commit delinquent acts to individual determinations to conform to social norms when Travis Hirschi (1969) publishes his work on the cause of delinquency. To explain why people adhere to rules, Hirschi identifies four types of social bonds. First is attachment: how a juvenile is tied to his or her parents, school, and peers. For instance, the parent-child bond is measured by the amount of time a child spends, the intimacy of communication he or she develops, and the affectional identification he or she has with his or her parents. Second is commitment: whether a juvenile aspires for educational attainment, vocational success, or achievements in other conventional lines of activity. Third is involvement: how much time and energy a youth invests in activities that promote the interests of society. The last bond is belief: whether a youth shares mainstream social beliefs and values that entail respect for law and order. Hirschi's social bonds theory remains a dominant paradigm in the social control literature. With his influential work, social control theory becomes more a theory of conformity than a theory of crime and its causation.

Outside the somewhat functionalist tradition that centers on socialization, personal control, social bonds, and conformity, there are a few unique perspectives worthy of notice in social control. Jack Gibbs (1981) defines social control as an attempt by one or more individuals to manipulate the behavior of another individual or individuals. In an interactionist perspective, he identifies five types of social control: referential, allegative, vicarious, modulative, and prelusive. Donald Black equalizes social control to "all of the practices by which people define and respond to deviant behavior" (1984: xi). Allan Horwitz (1990) develops a systematic typology of social control in terms of style, form, and effectiveness. Victor Shaw views social control as "any mechanism or practice for securing individual compliance, maintaining collective order and normative consistency, or dealing with problematic or deviant situations" (1996: 26). Analyzing the

Chinese work unit as an agent of social control, he explores the West versus the Third World, formal versus informal, primary versus secondary group, social versus organizational, regulative versus suggestive, and external versus internal dimensions of social control.

In substance use and abuse research, a universal assumption analogous to social control theory is that most people do not drink, smoke, or use illicit drugs because they are well regulated, controlled, and protected in biological, psychological, primary-group relational, communal, cultural, and social dimensions. Urie Bronfenbrenner (1977) proposes an ecological model, which later is expanded and refined by Jay Belsky (1993). According to the ecological model, there are four levels of influence on the individual's psychological development and social functioning. The ontogenetic denotes the individual and his or her personal characteristics such as physical features and personality traits. The microsystem refers to the individual's primary and secondary ties, including family, school, and peer groups, with which he or she spends the majority of time. The exosystem describes the neighborhood and community where the individual resides. And the macrosystem consists of cultural values, shared beliefs, economic events, and other social forces that have pervasive influence on the individual. At each level, there exist both protective factors that prevent the individual from maladjustment and risk factors that predispose the individual to problem behavior. At the ontogenetic level, Ralph Tarter and Michael Vanyukov (1994) put forth a liability model, suggesting that some individuals are born with a genetic vulnerability to developing alcohol use disorders. Risk factors for alcohol and drug abuse at the individual level may further include early onset of puberty, cognitive impairment, affective and behavioral dysregulation, temperament, sensation-seeking propensity, psychopathology, psychiatric disorder, coping and problem-solving skills deficits, and interpersonal skills deficits.

Similarly, factors contributing to the individual's alcohol and drug abuse in the microsystem may range from parental alcohol and/or drug use, family acceptance of alcohol and/or drug use, poor communication across the generational line, low cohesion among siblings, inconsistent and harsh discipline by parents or teachers, inadequate training and monitoring in school, and physical abuse and neglect by adult figures, to affiliation with delinquent peers. For instance, among conventional families, parents of at-risk adolescents are found to be not as successful as other parents in communicating their beliefs and values (Harbach and Jones 1995). When the family itself becomes dysfunctional, children are likely to experience problems in behavioral self-regulation, associate with delinquent peers, and therefore become a high risk for substance use and abuse (Dawes, Clark, Moss, Kirisci, and Tarter 1999). In the exosystem, risk factors may include crime, gang violence, drug dealing, poverty, inadequate housing, and lack of opportunities and resources across the neighborhood and community. Numerous studies point to the connection between crime and drug use in most inner-city areas and some ethnic enclaves (Bray and Marsden 1999). Finally, in the macrosystem, tolerance toward substance use, incorporation of substance use in cultural rituals and social functions, media glamorization, commercial advertisements, and formation of a drug subculture encourage and promote substance use among the populace. For example, a liberal attitude toward marijuana has made its use individualized. Marijuana use is now commonly found outside of the subcultural groups with which it was once associated. Some researchers hence argue that the practice needs to be studied at a personal level, as a practical, routine component of people's everyday lives (Hathaway 1997).

While substance use and abuse result from a lack or loss of control at various ecological levels, social reactions to the problem still call for nothing but control. Among the main measures of control are treatment, prevention, deterrence, border interdiction, and crop eradication (Fraser and Kohlert 1988). The U.S. drug policy that builds exactly upon these components, however, draws more criticisms than acclamations from both practice and research. Some charge that it is a result of moral panic; it is a weapon to further class interests; it is a criminalization of the threatening labor group by the higher-paid labor group; it is an agent for maintaining the stratification patterns of racial/ethnic minorities and women; and it is a targeted assault on the African American family (Hall 1997; Auerhahn 1999). Others suggest that the U.S. drug policy be reconstructed so that it emphasizes a community-up, rather than a social-planning, hierarchy-down, approach; it takes a communitarian perspective that recognizes the libertarian goal of personal freedom, the authoritarian concern for character, and the liberal desire to protect rights and promote welfare; it considers the interaction of the drug (agent), the person (host), and the cultural setting (environment); and it focuses on reducing harm, increasing safety, providing needed care, and seeking a balance between formal and informal control (Kleiman 1992–1993; Noguera and Morgan 1993–1994; Lewis, Duncan, and Clifford 1997).

THEORETICAL FRAMEWORK

The social control perspective posits that substance use is an intentional or unintentional escape from social control on the part of users. The questions then are: what is social control? How does an escape from social control take place? Why does an escape from social control possibly lead to substance use and abuse?

Definition

Control refers to either a state of affairs within one entity or a contrast of force between two parties. As a state of affairs, it means equilibrium, order, peace, and functionality of a system. As a contrast of force, it implies one part has more authority, power, and influence over the other in a confrontation, competition, or situation. For instance, when one says he or she is in control amid a wave of coughing after a deep inhalation of smoked tobacco, he feels he is capable of using his bodily power to accommodate the influence of tobacco intake and to swing back to his normal state where he thinks clearly and behaves responsibly.

Social control takes place in social contexts. It involves language, communications, religious beliefs, cultural norms, social customs, laws, and institutional restraints to keep people, groups, organizations, and communities where they are and doing what they are supposed to do in social interactions. From a functionalist perspective, a society maintains a proper level of social control when individual members and subsystems are well coordinated, regulated, and integrated in the whole system's function and evolution. From a critical point of view, however, an apparently viable social system often involves a relentless, oppressive, and exploitative application of social control by the rich, privileged, and powerful against the poor, disadvantaged, and powerless. As far as individuals are concerned, social control received from the outside affects self-control experienced inside.

The social control perspective applies the concept of social control to the field of substance use and abuse. From this perspective, people normally do not use substances because they are in control, under proper constraints from dominant social sources. Most people who use substances are capable of accommodating the effect of a limited amount of substance consumed as they tend to restore order and control, with appropriate guidance and restraints from positive social influences. A few people, however, use substances because they experience an improper level of control from conventional social agents. An improper level can be measured as either insufficient or excessive. Control can be analyzed either in the dimension of attachment, how an individual is tied to primary and secondary groups and institutions, or in the dimension of regulation, how an individual is guided by laws, social norms, common beliefs, and ethics. As substance use exacerbates, users move further away from conventional controls. Ironically, the void vacated by conventional controls is not the user's heaven for ultimate freedom. Instead, it immediately becomes the user's cage for total subjection to and absolute control by dependence, addition, and association with deviant subculture.

Theoretical Image

Control is a pervasive state within the individual. On the ontological level, one is subject to biological and psychological limits as to what and how much he or she can do at each moment and in his or her whole life.

As a social member, one takes on certain roles, associates with certain groups, participates in certain activities, follows different rules, and frames his or her daily routine in a structured way. One may retreat from active social life and become involved in nonproductive activities, such as drug use and vagrancy. But when one engages in a nonproductive life, one just enters into another world of rule and control. In drug use, controls from chemical dependency, psychological craving, drug dealers, peer users, and drug subcultures are often far more powerful than any or all conventional controls combined.

Control is a universal phenomenon in society. Individuals form groups. Groups make up organizations. Organizations operate in communities. Communities connect to each other by town, city, or county, which cluster into a state, and further a nation. While each individual entity develops its own internal governance, all social units in a larger system are usually subject to general legal, ideological, moral, linguistic, and bureaucratic controls imposed by the system. A particular social unit may fall under a state of "out of control." But when it does so, it may just become subjected to the control of some more powerful forces. For instance, a broken family where children become codependents to their father's alcoholism and mother's heroine addiction may be dialectically characterized as being totally controlled by the crushing power of substance and substance abuse.

Because a wide net of control is in place, most individuals do not use substances. Across families, ethnic groups, professional associations, work organizations, and governmental bureaucracies, substance use is not a major issue either. In cases when people use substances or where substance is used, there are identifiable problems in control. Specifically, individuals may use substances when they are not properly attached to their family, school, community, and other conventional agencies or when they are too closely associated with a problematic group or deviant subculture. Social groups may justify, promote, and protect substance use when they are not properly settled in the mainstream or when they are guided by some rebellious beliefs, ideas, and values. A society may adopt certain particular substances and witness certain levels of substance use when it is located in an isolated area or when it follows some age-old customs, practices, and rituals to preserve its culture and to maintain its relationship with nature. A historical era may feature a high, zero, or low level of use in certain or all substances when it goes through social disorganization, social transformation, general abstinence, or totalitarian control. The whole world may experience ups and downs in the variety and severity of substance use as social control loosens and tightens in its full spectrum of power and influence from time to time and from place to place. For instance, family runaways and school dropouts are more likely to use drugs than those youths who follow the footsteps of their middle-class parents and do adequate academic work in school; youth gangs and criminal groups are more likely to connive and use substances than sport clubs and professional associations; aboriginal societies in Pacific islands, remote mountainous regions, and near the North Pole are known to have adapted to the use of specific substances available in their unique environment; the United States attempted a national prohibition of alcohol in the first part of the twentieth century, while China was plagued with opium use during foreign invasions and civil wars from the Opium War in 1840 to the founding of the communist state in 1949; and across the globe, drug use is usually higher in affluent, liberal, democratic, Western, and capitalist nations than in indigent, conservative, authoritarian, Oriental, and socialist countries.

For the widely used substances, such as alcohol, tobacco, and caffeine, while their abuse can be traced to problems in social control, their regular use is apparently, though ironically, caused by the widespread and effective control of mass production, commercial media, trade, Western-style development, and bureaucratism. Alcohol, tobacco, and caffeine are produced, packaged, and shipped in large quantities from factories to retailers, from cities to rural areas, and from developed countries to developing societies. Consumption of name-brand alcohol, tobacco, and caffeine is portrayed by commercial media as a symbol of elegance, privilege, and success, in professional work and by Western-style development, while home brews, water pipes, and natural beverages are associated with tradition, frugality, and backwardness. In a bureaucratized working environment, having a cup of coffee during work, smoking a cigarette during the break, and drinking alcoholic beverages after hours seem to be just as natural and appropriate as wearing a suit, using a telephone, and keying a computer for business tasks and occasions.

Theoretical Components

The social control perspective examines how social control is related to substance use and abuse. Inherent in the perspective are five major theoretical components.

Source of Control

Sources of control vary in terms of where they originate, how they relate to the individual, what form they take, and how they exert their influences. First, there are external versus internal controls. External controls refer to controls from the outside, including parental discipline, rules and structured routines in school, legal codes, public opinion, law enforcement, criminal justice, and other social constraints. Internal controls include conscience, ego ideals, self-discipline, psychological rules, and physical limits. For instance, vomiting after consumption of alcohol may be the work of a self-adjustment mechanism activated when physical limits are threatened. External and internal controls are obviously interrelated. Conscience and self-discipline develop as the individual learns social mores and folkways through family and school. The effect of laws and social influences on an individual depends upon how broadly and deeply he or she internalizes external controls in his or her socialization process.

Second, primary controls come from parents, spouses, siblings, relatives, and kinship. Secondary controls are imposed by school, employment organizations, associations, community, and the government. While the former works by blood linkage, intimacy, example, and persuasion, the latter applies its power through formal sanction, such as reward and penalty. For example, parents may dissuade children from drug use by a show of love or a reference to family reputation whereas school, employer, association, or the government is likely to threaten drug users with expulsion, denial of employment, annulment of membership, or imprisonment.

Third, institutional sources include family, school, organizations, governmental agencies, and other entities with an identifiable structure. Contextual sources are mass media, public opinion, general sentiments, and overall social morale. Control by institutional sources may consist of various practical constraints through affiliation, physical arrangement, routinized structure, and regulated behavior. For instance, one drinks coffee because it is provided in the employee lounge by his or her employer or one gains no access to illegal drugs when he or she is incarcerated in a maximum-security prison. On the other hand, control from contextual sources takes place as long as one settles into an environment. He or she breathes the air, smells the odor, hears the voice, feels the sentiment, and gradually comes under the influence of the communal beliefs, values, and ways of thinking and acting. In the age of mass media, a number of people would change their attitude toward marijuana should media spread the word that marijuana is a useful agent in the treatment of AIDS and other diseases.

Finally, material controls target the body. They include medications, therapeutic devices, physical activities, and visible rewards. In narcotic treatment, addicts take medications to alleviate withdrawal symptoms and to maintain bodily functions. Spiritual controls, in contrast, act on the mind. They consist of message, information, knowledge, belief, and any other symbolism strongly felt by the recipient. Although spiritual controls are fluid and elusive in form, they can be highly penetrating and powerful in nature. In twelve-step or Alcoholics Anonymous meetings, participants work collectively to identify their shared weaknesses and strengths in confrontation with their commonly characterized menace, addiction or alcoholism. Generally, as science has established itself as the ultimate authority of knowledge, many people would drink wine regularly should science allege that it has proved the benefit of wine to health.

Dimension of Control

Control, in content, consists of two essential components. Attachment refers to the physical proximity an individual is tied to as well as the emotional investment he or she is engaged in with his or her source of control. There are voluntary and involuntary sides to attachment. On the voluntary side, one naturally or by choice lives with his or her family, goes to school, attends church, works in an organization, or becomes a professional or recreational member in an association. He or she takes a specific position, assumes a particular role, performs certain tasks, and participates in a variety of activities within the confines of the social unit to which he or she is attached. He or she spends time and energy to interact with other members, develop emotional contact with them, breed a sense of togetherness and belonging within the group, cultivate a communal concern for the welfare of the group, and become physically and emotionally integrated with the group. For example, family attachment involves all the elements of both physical presence and emotional investment. While it usually leads to a positive tradition within a family, such as a family of medical practice, professional achievements, or philanthropy, family attachment is also occasionally blamed for perpetuating crime, substance abuse, gambling, prostitution, welfare dependency, and other social vices across generations. The mafia family has long been a sensational phenomenon in media and literature. So has an alcoholic family in the medical circle.

Involuntary attachment occurs when one is forcibly taken into custody, being either locked up in a jail or incarcerated in a prison, being either restrained to a shock treatment procedure or confined to a mental hospital. To a lesser degree, involuntary attachment takes place when one is, by the requirement of law or the power of persuasion, recruited to a military training camp, a religious cult, a clandestine group, or a superstitious movement. In involuntary attachment, one may be required to follow a rigid routine, perform extraordinary deeds, and demonstrate his or her loyalty to the group or submission to the leader through physical exposure, endurance, and sacrifice. Among some secretive groups, members are sometimes initiated by drinking a large bowl of alcohol mixed with one another's blood. Some superstitious groups require their members to ritually swallow a dose of mixture specially prepared by their master. In American prisons, inmates are often exposed to underground drug dealing and drug use. Some of them develop a habit of smoking and drug use just through their association with the prison environment.

The other essential component of control is regulation. Regulation involves laws, values, beliefs, sentiments, and standards of evaluation that mold, shape, and guide people in their personality, thoughts, and behavior. There are formal and informal aspects of regulation. Formal regulation builds upon established laws, rules, and regulations, as well as their institutionalized sanctions. For example, retailers must fulfill certain requirements to deal alcohol and tobacco products. They can be fined if they operate a bar without a liquor license or sell cigarettes to minors. Marijuana, cocaine, and heroine are controlled substances in most countries. One can be charged with a crime and face specific punishment if found in possession, sales, or use of one of those substances.

Informal regulation, on the other hand, draws from the influence of traditions, customs, fashions, common beliefs, general values, and public sentiments. It works most of the time because the majority of people follow folkways and overall social expectations in their drive toward peer recognition, professional success, and self-actualization. It loses its effect sometimes because a few who fail to observe informal rules do not face any obvious penalty other than some embarrassment or inconvenience. For instance, one may only receive a few strange-looking eye contacts when he or she lights a cigarette in a meeting room where no sign of smoking prohibition is posted. In a group to which one is closely attached, however, influence from sources of informal regulation can be gradually penetrating and long-lasting. For example, a father's liberal attitude toward drug use may sink well into the mind of his children, becoming a catalyst for drug use and abuse.

Degree of Control

By common sense, there exists either control or no control. Problems arise when a situation is out of control or there is no control. The control perspective challenges the simplistic view held by the general public about social control. It places social control in a continuum and aims to examine the various consequences of differential degrees of control on an individual's behavior in general and substance use in particular.

The degree of control in the normal range is characterized as proper control. Proper control features appropriate attachment and adequate regulation. With appropriate attachment, individuals develop meaningful connections to family, kinship, school, church, employer, interest-based association, community, and other social institutions. They play different roles, perform different tasks, and engage in routine interactions with parents, siblings, relatives, classmates, teachers, fellow church-goers, co-workers, supervisors, people of the same occupation or interest, neighbors, community activists, local leaders, and other social actors. When it comes to achievement, reward, and honor, they have someone and somewhere to celebrate together, to thank, and to share with. When it comes to failure, penalty, and dishonor, they have someone and somewhere to turn to for consolation, encouragement, and advice. Individuals therefore maintain a good sense of coherence, belonging, and togetherness in their social life.

By adequate regulation, individuals grow with positive socialization experiences. They internalize linguistic rules, religious beliefs, cultural norms, social customs, legal codes, and other social conventions. They understand what is appropriate, acceptable, good, right, legal, and conventional and avoid what is inappropriate, unacceptable, bad, wrong, illegal, and unconventional. For example, a teenager automatically turns away from alcohol when he believes use of alcohol is not appropriate for a youth of his age. He turns away from controlled substances when he knows use of controlled substances is illegal. He feels a sense of embarrassment, shame, or guilt for whoever breaks laws or conventions regarding substance use and other acts.

Out of the normal range are either excessive or insufficient controls. Excessive control manifests in intense attachment and severe regulation. Under intense attachment, individuals are overly tied to social groups so that they do not have much personal space for themselves. They spend most of their time and energy on the activities dictated by group leaders within group enclaves. They work for their groups and do whatever their groups call them to do, including substance use, violence, and self-sacrifice. For instance, military servicemen and -women are required to take certain substances when they enter into a battlefield with a highly anticipated use of chemical or biological weapons by enemy troops. More pointedly, young people who turn to gang groups as their alternatives for a sense of belonging may make steady strides toward substance use, violence, and criminal behavior under a high level of coherence with peers and leaders within the gangs.

Severe regulation occurs when an individual succumbs to the restrictive rules and highly structured routines imposed by a group to which he or she is intensely attached. Generally, it takes place in a time when there is a heightened level of surveillance, discipline, and control over people's thoughts and acts or in a place where mass media sound restrictive, political order becomes oppressive, and legal system turns punitive. At the individual level, severe regulation takes effect when one is unduly influenced by a type of belief, value, ideology, philosophy, or practice. He first learns about his source of influence by accident, curiosity, excessive exposure, or long-term contact. But once he decides on an attitude toward it, he takes that attitude to his heart, subjecting his thoughts and acts to its control and influence. For instance, one picks up the drug legalization argument from mass media, through exposure to a subculture, or by influence of his or her significant others. He later becomes so identified with it that he risks his health, wealth, and legal standing to practice and advocate for it.

Insufficient control lies in loose attachment and lax regulation. Loose attachment to social groups puts individuals in a state of floating over reality. They feel lonely and alienated because they do not coherently belong to any group and have difficulty participating in social activities. They feel a sense of aimlessness and meaninglessness in their life because they do not have any reference group to compare nor any significant companions to share what they do and have accomplished. To the extreme, a few individuals may retreat from active social life and become nonproductive through alcohol abuse and drug addiction.

Lax regulation leads individuals to a lack or loss of guidance in their thoughts and behavior. They are uncertain and confused because they do not learn important moral concepts and have difficulty distinguishing what is right from what is wrong. They often struggle in a state of anomie, chaos, or inaction because they are out of touch with effective social norms, because they are preoccupied with some defunct beliefs and values, or because they receive conflicting rules from their environment. In the most polarized situation, some individuals feel nothing works and anything goes. Under this sentiment, they loosen their internal restraints and indulge in drunkenness, hallucination, dependency, or anarchism.

Substitution of Control

Problems in social control may lead to substance use and abuse. But use of substances does not provide individuals with immunity from control. In fact, as use escalates into abuse and dependency, control may become an ever-salient issue for individuals to deal with in their daily life. In a sense, various influences of substance and substance use experienced by individuals can be viewed as natural substitutes for normal controls they struggle to loosen or disconnect from social agents.

First, as individuals keep using a substance, they experience a lesser effect of the substance. In order to maintain a same level of effect, they have to increase the dosage of its intake. The phenomenon is identified as tolerance. It is generally perceived as the body's ability to compensate for the chemical imbalance caused by a substance. From a control point of view, however, it is the body's submission or adaptation to the onslaught of the substance. The control conceptualization makes sense especially in light of physical dependence. Physical dependence is defined by the occurrence of a withdrawal syndrome, a collection of symptoms that occur when the level of a substance drops in the system. For instance, heroin users develop tolerance to heroin. When they stop taking it abruptly, they soon experience running nose, chills, fever, diarrhea, and other painful symptoms. Fearful of its withdrawal syndrome, addicts keep using the substance and therefore continue their subjection to the power of its control.

Second, some substances do not produce apparently dramatic and medically well-defined physical withdrawal syndromes. But still users tend to use those substances frequently, sometimes toward an ever-increasing intensity, develop a habit of use or establish a behavioral pattern of dependency, crave substances when not using them for a certain duration, and relapse after a period of forcible or voluntary abstinence. The phenomenon is referred to as psychological dependency. Besides those substances that are known to be mainly associated with psychological dependency, such as marijuana, amphetamine, and cocaine, psychological dependency also applies to the substances that cause physical dependence. In view of control, psychological dependence reflects the mind's obedience and subjection to the forcible influence of a substance.

Third, between body and mind, substance use and abuse may result in improper attachment of mind to body and improper regulation of mind over body. Improper means either insufficient or excessive. On the one extreme, users light a pipe, take an injection, and bear other substance-related physical challenges in disregard to the beliefs, attitudes, sentiments, feelings, moods, or senses of privilege, decency, and dignity held in their own mind. On the other extreme, they follow a propaganda, advocacy, hearsay, misinformation, vogue, fantasy, or superstition to take an unusual amount of a substance without any concern for the forbearance, endurance, health, and well-being of their own body. At an abstract level, improper controls between body and mind following substance use and abuse can be properly perceived as substitutions of natural control mechanisms by substance influences or interferences.

Finally, upon substance use and abuse, individuals network with other users, establish relationships with sources of supply, gather use-related information, and develop patterns of use in terms of time, location, and ritual. As they proceed on those fronts, they gradually come under the association as well as influence of various substance use individuals, groups, agents, arguments, and ideologies. They may also run into the mighty control machinery of drug war and criminal justice. At some point in time, substance users may still have to experience a significant level of control from many nonetheless social sources, although in a way often different from the normal and the conventional.

Restoration of Control

While individuals may indeed experience a considerable amount of control during substance use and abuse by way of substitution, various social agents normally only recognize a loosened, disturbed, or disrupted control they face with substance-affected subjects. They naturally make efforts to restore the control they enjoy over the individuals to the normal level.

There are many social agents concerned with substance use and substance users. Although most of them have the intent to restore control and order, not all of them achieve a restorative consequence of their restoration efforts. The government, the criminal justice system, and the conservative alliance often, though inadvertently, push substance users further into abuse, addiction, dependency, deviance, and criminality by shaming them, demonizing them, depriving them of their properties or rights, imprisoning them, or isolating them. Obviously, negative punishment does not always teach people a lesson about the positive effect of law and bring them back to compliance with the law. Alternatives are therefore explored as truth fails to bear out the age-old proposition that two negatives (a negative reaction, such as punishment, to a negative situation, such as substance abuse) make one positive (a restoration of order or a rehabilitation of a drug addict).

Among nonpenal reactions to substance use and abuse are medical treatment, harm reduction, family therapy, group sessions, vocational training, counseling, and therapeutic communities. Although they are ideologically different from negative penal control, they are conceptually in line with it as other styles of control, either conciliatory, compensatory, therapeutic, or restorative. Specifically, medical treatment is to restore biochemical equilibrium or a proper level of attachment and regulation between body and mind. Harm reduction is to reach out to substance users, to extend social support to them, and to raise their self-concern for health. It aims to compensate substance users for some of the loss they sustain in the acquisition of essential knowledge and values about human survival and physical well-being. It also represents a conciliatory gesture from the social mainstream: we do not blame you for what you do, so come back to our embrace for a sense of care and support. Family therapy and group sessions are to reestablish attachment to primary and secondary social institutions and to reactivate their regulation over individuals. Vocational training is to introduce the discipline of work and to routinize individual behavior in accordance with task performance. Finally, counseling, self-help, and therapeutic communities often involve a particular religious belief or ideological argument to create a new view of the world, to rebuild self-control, and to legitimize a communal living arrangement that provides substance users with a structure for their daily life.

Theoretical Applications

The control perspective relates the object of study to its internal forces as well as to its external environment. By examining how it remains in a normal state of control, it sheds light on why it deviates from the norm when problems arise in its internal and external control mechanisms.

With regard to substance users, the control perspective draws attention to the relationships they have with family, school, community, and various other conventional institutions. Is substance use attributable to any one of those relationships? What relationship is primarily responsible? What major problem is there in the relationship? Is it a problem in attachment: are they properly tied to various social agencies so that they have the opportunity to participate in social activities, demonstrate their social worthiness, and develop a sense of belonging? Is it a problem in regulation: are they properly guided by norms and rules prevailing in mainstream social agencies so that they have the motivation to follow socially appropriate attitudes as well as the opportunity to maintain a sense of direction in their daily life? Is it a problem of insufficient or excessive control? What substitute is there for a damaged relationship with a dysfunctional social institution? For example, young people may join gang groups or become identified with a deviant subculture amid the void of support from family. If no obvious problems exist in the relationships with various social institutions, is one of those social institutions itself a source of influence for substance use? It is natural that children follow the footsteps of parents in alcohol use, students model after teachers or classmates in smoking, and workers synchronize with colleagues in consumption of caffeine. The same holds true for illegal drug use. Finally, when substance is used, how much are individual users controlled by the power of substance, casual use, recreational use, habitual use, dependent use, problem use, abuse, or addiction? What control ensues from society, medical treatment, group therapy, professional counseling, vocational training, police arrest, property confiscation, or imprisonment?

Regarding a particular substance, the control perspective is interested in examining its chemical structure and pharmaceutical properties to explain the nature and degree of control it has over its individual users. Why does it cause tolerance? Why does it result in withdrawal symptoms? How does it relate to psychological craving? Does use lead to permanent or temporary change to the neurochemical system? From a sociological point of view, the control perspective studies various images, fears, and control measures developed and instituted toward a substance. Are those images, fears, and control measures scientifically, objectively, and fairly based upon the substance's natural properties? What historical events or social forces are there to shape the formation of a particular characterization of or legal action toward a particular substance? Specifically, what control status does it have under current law? Is it a regulated product: only licensed retailers are allowed to sell it to people of a certain age or only physicians are authorized to prescribe it to people with certain diagnosed ailments? Is it a controlled substance? Is possession, dealing, or use of it subject to legal sanctions? Are there any irrationalities in legal sanctions against the substance? What change is necessary and possible to its current control status?

As far as control and control agents are concerned, the control perspective looks into their respective nature, process, degree, and change in both pre- and postuse periods. Is control rational, balanced, and effective? Is it restorable when it is disturbed by substance use? What does it take to restore control? Similarly, are control agents reasonable and supportive or punitive and repressive? What approach does each control agent take toward substance use in particular and deviance in general: forgive, condemn, or punish? Are control agents willing and able to mend a relationship strained by substance use? For instance, harsh discipline by parents may lead to rebellion from children. Rebellious youth may engage in smoking and illegal drug use to challenge the control by their parents. When parents take harsher actions to punish their wayward children, they may make their relationship with children even more difficult to repair and improve. The vicious cycle applies more saliently to more dominant social control agencies, such as the police, the court, and the corrections. Users of controlled substances are not only punished as lawbreakers, but also cast out from the mainstream society by an officially kept record of law violations.

Empirical Tests

The control perspective focuses on various social control agencies and their respective influence on individual behavior. While qualitative methods can be applied to identify and verify different sources, types, forms, and styles of control, quantitative methods can be employed to measure the degree of intimacy, intensity, or effectiveness pertaining to a specific control and control relationship.

Specifically, case studies are useful for gaining detailed knowledge about individual substances, substance users, and control agents. For a particular substance, research can be done to measure its control effect on the human body and mind, document its control status over time and across national borders, and ascertain its current control status in terms of morality, legality, and rationality. Regarding individual users, representative cases can be identified to study how people are normally related to family, school, employment organization, interest-based association, community, and governmental agency; how a strained relationship people have with one social control agent may impact their relationships with other control sources; what range of problems people may get into in both self-control and social control; how problems in social control are differentially associated with substance use; what control people fear and feel they lose following substance use; what effort users make to restore control; what pressure they face from conventional social control institutions to terminate substance use; and how likely they come back to their normal relationships with various social control agents. Finally, each social control agent can be examined in its influence, positive or negative, strong or weak, supportive or punitive, across different phases of substance use, prevention, initiation, escalation, habituation, addiction, treatment, and recovery. For example, school can serve as a strong positive source of influence for drug prevention. It may also become a negative, though weak, test ground for drug use among youth. When drug use takes place, school tends to be punitive rather than supportive: drug-using youths are suspended or expelled rather than treated or helped.

Historical analysis is indispensable to linking the change in moral and legal discourses to the use of substance over time. In the time of high morality and tight control, how do family, school, community, and other social institutions each play their due roles? How are they all integrated into a functional social system to keep people in line? How are individuals socialized into the mainstream so that they follow positive social norms and values in their behavior? What measures are instituted to control the production, transport, and use of substances? How are drug use and abuse shamed, condemned, and penalized? What level of drug use and abuse is recorded? Likewise, studies can be conducted to portray and assess social control agencies, substance classification systems, public opinions, deviant subcultures, civil rights movements, and their respective effect on substance use and abuse, in the time of low morality and loosened control. Historical analysis may also be combined with case studies to catalog the course of change for individual substances and social control agents in relation to substance use and users.

Survey research has been essential to establishing, validating, and refuting major arguments pertaining to social control theories (Hirschi 1969; Krohn and Massey 1980; Agnew 1985). By face-to-face, telephone, or mail interview, sensible questions can be designed to measure various social control agents, substance use and abuse, deviant and criminal behaviors, and other important variables. With survey data, cross-sectional relations between social bonds and substance use can be ascertained. Change in social control, substance use, and their mutual influence may also be catalogued through longitudinal design and analysis. For instance, regulation through family disciplines and substance use can be surveyed in different periods to measure their respective change as well as the overall trend in their correlations. Survey interviews as individual research methods are important techniques in both case studies and historical analysis.

Experimental studies are applicable in empirical tests for the control perspective as well. In fact, a number of social projects have been implemented through experimental design to put social control theories into practice. Some of those projects target family and school, such as PATHE (Positive Action Through Holistic Education) and a parenting training program in Seattle, while others line up with community-wide organizations. The intent is the same: strengthening conventional systems to increase their influence in a youth's life. From a research point of view, experimental design can be used to ascertain causal relationships between social control and substance use. For example, an educational series on drug use for parents is introduced as experimental conditions to one group while it is withheld from a comparable group in terms of all relevant variables. Attitudes toward drugs and actual drug use can be measured and compared before and after experimental conditions among both parents and children to see if parents willingly and effectively pass on their natural values and learned messages to their children.

POLICY IMPLICATIONS

The control perspective relates substance use to different forces of control in individual life. In policy arenas, it provides directions and strategies for decision makers and practitioners in various concerned fields to effectively deal with substance use and abuse as challenging social problems.

Public Health

Medical researchers and practitioners study biochemical and neurobiological conditions among substance users. To understand those conditions, they sometimes delve into users' genetic structure and attribute use to heredity. To develop medical treatment, they often begin with the normal biochemical equilibrium among human beings and figure out how to restore a disturbed system to its normal balance for substance users. From a control point of view, genetic influences take effect along with the social functioning of family: the closer one is tied to his or her family and the more effectively one is regulated by his or her family rules, the more family influence one experiences in his or her thoughts and acts and the more hereditary traits researchers are able to identify in genetic research. In diagnosis, the control perspective may guide medical professionals to assess the severity of use and abuse by the degree of control lost between the body and mind. Medical treatment may therefore be approached as a restoration of order and equilibrium by appropriate substitutes of control. As a general reference in practice, an index of control may be established for users, substances, and treatment medications. For instance, users are identified by the amount of control they may lose due to substance use, substances by the potential of control they may exert over users, and treatment medications by the degree of control they may restore for users.

Health service professionals, including health educators, counselors, and prevention workers, raise awareness about health lifestyles in the general public or work on specific health problems faced by special at-risk groups. The control perspective can obviously benefit them in various unique ways. First, it highlights the importance of mass media, social perceptions, and cultural atmosphere in influencing individual thoughts and behaviors. Educational messages about health risks and hazards, when they are sent naturally through various social sources, can be more powerful than when they are imposed forcibly upon people by the government in the form of public campaigns. Second, the control perspective affirms the power of conventional institutions in socializing people and engaging them in positive social activities. Health service professionals need to work closely with family, school, employers, and community organizations in substance use prevention and intervention. Third, problems often come from conventional sources of control as they play a significant role in individual life. Health service professionals need to identify negative sources of influence, analyze excessiveness or insufficiency in attachment and regulation, and work to restore balance with appropriate control substitutes. For example, it may be a challenge to counsel a youth who grows up with an excessive attachment to his or her drug-using parents or an excessive regulation by his or her parents' liberal attitudes toward drug use.

Social Control

The drug war views drug use as a social menace. It has dramatically radicalized social control reactions toward drug use and drug users. With the social control perspective, a diverse yet balanced approach can be taken toward various issues concerning substance use.

First, substance use does not boil down to drug use. In fact, it is the use of a variety of substances that provides a general background for hard-drug use. Social control therefore should begin with general substance use, including drinking, smoking, medication, and use of all potentially addictive substances. Second, social control does not equalize elimination and punishment. It also includes public education, promotion of a healthy lifestyle, mass media, social bonds offered by various conventional institutions, professional counseling, group help, medical treatment, and social support. Third, social control agents do not involve only police officers, prosecutors, and prison guards. There are more influential participants in the process: parents, teachers, peers, co-workers, supervisors, role models, service professionals, medical personnel, community leaders, and governmental officials. Fourth, between supply and demand, the social control perspective focuses more on demand. Once demand is reduced or eliminated, supply will automatically die down. To control demand is mainly to build strong family and school ties in the community, and to cultivate positive attitudes and lifestyles among individuals. Fifth, between substance use and substance users, the social control perspective pays more attention to users. While substance can be regulated through a range of control measures, from classification, licensing, legal restriction, substitution, and prohibition, to total elimination, users need and deserve far more care, service, guidance, and support during use, addiction, withdrawal, treatment, recovery, and return to society.

Finally, the social control perspective remains sensitive to the degree of attachment individuals have with different social institutions as well as the degree of regulation they are subject to by various social conventions. It warns against not only insufficiency but also excessiveness in attachment and regulation as possible causes of substance-related problems. It especially alerts the criminal justice system in its punitive intervention in substance possession, dealing, use, misuse, and abuse.

Life and Community

Substance use takes place in the community of life. Preventing substance use calls for the collective effort of the community. Treating addiction needs cooperative support from parents, siblings, relatives, and neighbors. Restoring normal life to people who are involved in substance abuse or misuse requires that proper sources of attachment and regulation be created and maintained in the community.

Specifically, the control perspective emphasizes the importance of family in individual life. While most families provide positive social bonds for their members, neglect, abuse, spoiling, restriction, and inconsistent disciplining are common familial causes for attention seeking, rebellion, deviation, and substance abuse by young children. To prevent substance use among youth, a strong family needs to be built so that parents interact closely, smoothly, and routinely with children to serve as their friends, mentors, role models, and sources of inspiration, guidance, and support. Second, the control perspective realizes the influence of school in individual development. School is where young people learn knowledge, develop skills, internalize rules and norms, and build social networks. It may also become a place where they are exposed to antisocial attitudes, associate with gangsters, and become disappointed, stressed out, and alienated. For example, high rates of substance use, mental disorder, and suicide are recorded among college students, partly because they suffer from a lack of attachment as they leave home to manage life on their own, and partly because they face the challenge of survival as they enter the classroom to compete for academic success. Professional counseling and positive social grouping are therefore needed to guide and support young people through their educational experience. Third, the control perspective points to the functional role of the neighborhood in fostering a collective spirit among residents. In a closely knit neighborhood, people keep eyes on each other's children and properties so that deviant behavior is kept in check and criminal victimization is deterred and prevented. In contrast, substance use and criminal activities may become rampant in a socially disorganized neighborhood where gang members fight for dominance, drug dealers make transactions in parks and on streets, and neighbors remain suspicious and hostile against each other. Reinventing neighborhood is not only important in providing a positive communal environment for residents, but also essential to building strong families, schools, and other grassroots institutions.

Finally, the control perspective views community as the place to resolve problems when they arise. Human beings are creative beings. While most people are law-abiding citizens, there are always a few outliers who tend to deviate from normal ways of thinking and acting. Life is a dynamic process. While people remain under control for most of their life, they may lose control sometimes on some matters. It is important to examine the source, the nature, the process, and the change of control an individual experiences in his or her life. By tradition, however, loss of control is simply condemned, shamed, and punished. In convention, people who have lost control are just shamed, distanced, and isolated. Most systematically, the criminal justice system has been established in the modern state to take deviants and criminals out of mainstream circulation for reform, rehabilitation, and punishment. Recognizing the alienating effect of punitive control and the importance of social bonds, the control perspective suggests that substance users and legal violators related to substance use be treated and helped in the community, with all necessary resources from family, relative networks, school, and neighborhood associations or organizations therein.

Work and Organization

Work presents a task in which individuals invest time and energy to demonstrate their talents, realize their potential, and create certain deeds of worth and pride. Employment organizations provide a framework by which individuals routinize their daily schedule, interact with people, evaluate their activities, and develop a sense of belonging. In the spirit of the control perspective, work and organizations are important sources of control for all working individuals.

There is a wide spectrum of work and organizations in terms of their control over individuals. In the East as well as in socialist countries, companies or work units not only supervise workers during their time at work, but also monitor their marriage, friendship, hobbies, and other life-related activities. In contrast, Western as well as capitalist employers or corporations are primarily interested in what employees do during their contract time with the company. They generally do not bother to know where and how employees live their private life outside the working hours. Regarding illicit drug use, a socialist work unit may condemn its drug-using employees and force them into treatment, whereas a capitalist employer may take no action on the matter as long as its employees do their assigned work and pose no danger to its profit-making business.

From the control perspective, both excessive and insufficient attachment to and regulation by work organizations can put employees at risk for substance use in particular and deviant behavior in general. In contemporary society, since most people work and working people spend most of their activity time on work-related tasks, employment organizations have a significant role to play in shaping individuals' thoughts and influencing their behaviors. Specifically, corporate culture may promote or prevent substance use. Various prevailing conceptions and images about substance use are currently associated with corporate culture: a cup of coffee at work, fine wines at business banquets, corporate executives lighting up a cigar while presiding over a business meeting, professional women holding a smoke-swirling cigarette outside downtown high-rise buildings at lunchtime, millionaire business owners gaining access to high-quality drugs in their secluded resorts, and children of business moguls or tycoons abusing drugs. To reverse the trend, sports, adventures, healthy lifestyles, and other alternatives have to be explored and promoted as sites and symbols for money, success, and pride. Second, work rules and company policies may deter or protect substance use. For instance, drug screening can effectively prevent employees from using controlled substances, whereas provision of coffee, smoking areas, and employee lounges may increase consumption of licit substances by employees. Also, stringent requirements on task performance may lead to substance use and abuse as employees struggle to manage their stress at work. Third, work organizations may shun or serve as sources of support for substance-using employees in treatment and recovery. Employers usually fire employees who experience problems in substance use or at best put them on unpaid leave. They seldom realize that they can sponsor programs to assist their drug-dependent employees toward recovery. For instance, a smoking-cessation group among co-workers within a company may work successfully upon peer pressure and organizational mandates. In China, some large-scale work units in drug-plagued areas even venture into providing comprehensive drug treatment services for their drug-dependent members.

In all, the control perspective views substance, substance use, and substance users in light of control. Substance, by its chemical composition and pharmaceutical properties, demonstrates different degrees of control over the human body and mind. Substance use, in terms of its cause, prevalence, and consequence, features a change of control among individuals and in society. People normally do not use substances when they are in control. A few may use substances when they experience excessive or insufficient attachment to or regulation by social institutions and their various norms. Society differs in moral, sentimental, and legal controls over individuals and substances. Substance use may run out of control when people are not properly guided in their thoughts and behaviors or social regulations of substances become irrational and unreasonable. On the part of substance users, involvement in substance use may begin with problems in personal or social control, either excessive or insufficient attachment to social groupings, excessive or insufficient regulation by social norms, or a proper attachment to and regulation by a group or subculture that features deviant or antisocial attitudes and behaviors. During substance use, users do not necessarily experience a lack of control. Instead, they are likely to face a variety of substitutes of control, from chemical dependency to subjection to drug subculture, from law enforcement intervention to treatment by medical professionals.

The control perspective sheds new light on the critical social issue of substance use and abuse. With the perspective, social control and its various sources, sites, dimensions, degrees, consequences, substitutes, and restoration options can be identified and examined to inform and enhance prevention and intervention in both general policy and specific strategies or tactics.

—7—

The Social Disorganization Perspective

Substance is used by individuals who live in particular neighborhoods, racial/ethnic enclaves, communities, and societies as well as over specific historical periods. Events that happen in the environment during their lifetime affect individuals in their attitudes and behavior toward substances. Change in the environment, especially when it takes place rapidly in a short period of time, can easily lead to value confusion, belief disorientation, and loss of normative control, prompting individuals to engage in substance use as their perceived mechanisms of avoidance, relief, or coping.

The social disorganization perspective follows substance users to their living era and environment. On the one hand, it examines why individuals move from one environment to another, how they struggle to adjust to a new environment, and how they are lured or forced into substance use, deviance, or criminal activity in the face of difficulty from the new environment or due to their individual misadjustment. On the other hand, it studies how a particular environment changes from generation to generation, how drastic change in a specific environment causes stress, disillusion, and disorder among individuals who live in it, and why substance use, deviance, crime, and other social problems tend to increase in a time when or in a place where change occurs abruptly.

SOURCES OF INSPIRATION

The idea of social disorganization springs out of the minds of sociologists at the University of Chicago in the 1920s. Following rapid industrialization and extensive urbanization at the turn of the century as well as in the aftermath of World War I, there seem to be omnipresent manifestations of unprecedented changes in the vast landscape of the United States. With financial and political support from the business elite of the nation and the city, Chicago sociologists come to grapple with the challenges of studying social change and providing the emerging middle class of managerial professionals with factual knowledge to technically and efficiently direct the course of change toward stability.

W. I. Thomas is the first scholar to conceptualize the problem of disorganization. Although he himself was forced to leave the University of Chicago in 1918, the intellectual seed planted by him soon germinated into a full-blown theoretical perspective, bringing an unprecedented preeminence to the Department of Sociology on campus. On the qualitative side, Chicago scholars rely upon observations, interviews, and personal documents to explore the meaning of life as experienced by people in the time or under an environment of social disorganization. W. I. Thomas and Florian Znaniecki (1920) examined various types of bowing or greeting letters, from ceremonial, informing, sentimental, and literary, to business letters, written by Polish immigrants in America and their relatives in Poland. They found that immigrants live in a world devoid of secure normative standards, not only because they have difficulty assimilating the norms and values of their new social environments, but also because what used to work for them in their rural communities of a different cultural tradition no longer serves their new needs of living in the midst of industrializing U.S. cities. Caught in the lack of normative guidance between their old and new worlds, immigrants develop an "anything goes, nothing works" attitude. With that attitude, they can easily drift into deviance, delinquency, divorce, mental disorder, and other forms of unruly behavior.

Thomas and Znaniecki's study of Polish peasants in Europe and America provides a classic statement of the social disorganization perspective. Using similar and other fieldwork methods, Chicago scholars venture into different dynamics of social disorganization to illustrate "the process by which the authority and influence of an earlier culture and system of social control are undermined and eventually destroyed" (Park, Burgess, and McKenzie 1967: 107). Thomas (1923) himself examined the life of a prostitute in *The Unadjusted Girl*. Nels Anderson (1923) studied homelessness in *The Hobo: The Sociology of the Homeless Man*. Ernest Mowner (1927) analyzed disorganized families in *Family Disorganization*. Louis Wirth (1928) and Harvey Zorbaugh (1929) focused on slums in their respective works *Ghetto* and *Gold Coast and Slum*. Frederich Thrasher (1927) researched gangs and gang activities in *The Gang*. Clifford Shaw (1930) followed the story of a delinquent boy in *The Jack Roller*. He later cooperated with Maurice Moore (1931) in *The Natural History of a Delinquent Career* and James McDonald (1938) in *Brothers in Crime*. Other scholars who concentrated on the "seamy side" of city life in the perspective of social disorganization include: Paul Cressey (1932) in *The Taxi-Dance Hall*, Norman Hayner (1936) in *Hotel Life*, and Edwin Sutherland (1937) in *The Professional Thief*.

While being strong and persistent in their internal-subjective approaches, Chicago scholars also emphasize efforts to objectively measure external factors and forces that affect both the process and the consequence of social disorganization. Robert Park (1936), in cooperation with Ernest Burgess, developed an ecological model to capture the interrelationships of people and their environment. Specifically, Park and Burgess divided the city into natural urban areas and focused on area characteristics for explanations of deviance, crime, and other social disorganization problems. For the city of Chicago, they identified five concentric zones, each of which has its own unique structure, organizations, inhabitants, and cultural features. At the center is the downtown business district occupied by commercial establishments, law and government offices, and business headquarters. At the outer reaches of the city is the commuter zone of satellite towns and suburbs inhabited by people with bountiful social, spatial, and economic resources. In between are the transition zone, the zone of workingmen's homes, and the residential zone. The zone of workingmen's homes provides blue-collar workers with close access to jobs and city transportation networks. The residential zone features single-family homes owned by small entrepreneurs, professionals, and managerial personnel. The zone in transition, however, gathers poor and unskilled beggars, bums, vagabonds, and other rootless people in dilapidated tenements next to old factories, warehouses, and red-light businesses. Being constantly pushed by the growing business district, it bears and exemplifies most of the bruises and wounds of urban social change: delinquency, school truancy, prostitution, gambling, substance abuse, mental illness, suicide, and adult crime.

The ecological model soon becomes the hallmark of the social disorganization perspective. Applying the model, Clifford Shaw and Henry McKay developed an analysis of the ecological distribution of delinquency. They first, along with their colleagues Frederick Forgaugh and Leonard Cottreel, examined 55,998 juvenile court records from 1900 to 1933 in the city of Chicago (1929). They then extended their analysis to cities in other parts of the nation (1969). The major findings they generalized from their research include: (a) delinquency is differently distributed throughout the city; (b) delinquency, along with other community problems, such as infant mortality, truancy, and mental disorders, occurs mostly in the areas nearest the central business zone; (c) areas of high delinquency are characterized by a high percentage of immigrants, a high percentage of nonwhites, a high percentage of families on relief, and a low percentage of home ownership;

and (d) some areas consistently suffer from high delinquency, regardless of the ethnic composition of the residents. Similarly, Robert Faris and Warren Dunham (1939) mapped the ecological distribution of public hospitalization for serious mental disorders. According to them, "the highest rates for schizophrenia are in hobohemia, the rooming-house, and foreign-born communities close to the center of the city... as these communities represent areas of some disorganization due to their close proximity to the steel factories" (Faris and Dunham 1939: 95).

Social disorganization theorizing continues after the Chicago School era. First are area studies conducted by Bernard Lander (1954) in Baltimore, Maryland; David Bordua (1959) in Detroit, Michigan; and Roland Chilton (1964) in Indianapolis, Indiana. Despite individual differences, all three studies show that ecological conditions, such as substandard housing, low income, and unrelated people living together, predict a high incidence of delinquency. Through the 1970s, while facing serious challenges for its validity in developed social contexts (Kornhauser 1978), the social disorganization theory found its vitality in the study of deviance in developing countries. Kirson Weinberg (1976) examined juvenile delinquency in Accra, Ghana. He found that delinquent youths are concentrated in areas characterized by physical deterioration, disintegration of traditional family structures, poor education, unskilled labor, poverty, alcoholism, and high rates of adult crime. Marshall Clinard and Daniel Abbott (1976) studied property crime in Kampala, Uganda. Comparing radically different rates of property offenses in two physically similar slums, they discovered that the low-crime slum has greater homogeneity in population, more family stability, a larger degree of sharing in tribal customs, more intimate interactions among residents, and a higher level of participation in community organizations. The inference from the study that normative control is critical in maintaining neighborhood coherence takes Marshall Clinard back from developing countries to developed societies. In *Cities with Little Crime: The Case of Switzerland*, Clinard (1978) reasoned that the low crime rate in the country is due to the tight normative organization bolstered by political decentralization, local responsibility, gradual urbanization, and generational integration across Swiss society. Also in a Western context, Richard Sollenberger (1968) invoked disorganization imagery to explain why children in Chinatown, the tightly knit, family-oriented Chinese-American enclave, do not become delinquents. Raymond Michalowski (1977) followed social and criminal patterns of urban traffic fatalities. He found that people involved in vehicular homicide tend to be those who are bombarded with marital trouble, emotional turmoil, loss of employment, and alcohol abuse in their traditionally disorganized ecological zones.

Interest in ecological conditions revives among criminologists in the 1980s and 1990s. Shifting from the traditional emphasis on value conflict, the new generation of social ecologists focus more on the association of community deterioration and economic decline to criminality (Byrne and Sampson 1985). Among various physical, economic, and social conditions examined are abandoned buildings, deserted houses, apartments in poor repair, trash and litter, graffiti, boarded-up storefronts, noise, congestion, lack of employment, limited job opportunities, population turnover, poverty concentration, and life cycles in community change. For instance, Ralph Taylor and Jeanette Covington (1988) followed the life cycle in urban areas, from increase in population density to change in racial or ethnic makeup to population thinning, and from building dwellings to residential decline or decay to housing replacement and upgrade or neighborhood gentrification. They pointed out that community fear and crime rates increase when urban areas undergo such cyclical change (1993). To a lesser degree though, social ecologists also look into the nonmaterial dimension of disorganized neighborhoods. Along with community fear, siege mentality, poverty concentration effect, and social altruism are conceptualized to explain why crime and social problems spread, persist, or decrease in response to prevalent sentiments shared by residents in the community (Wilson 1987; Anderson 1990; Chamlin and Cochran 1997; Holloway 1998).

Studies on substance and substance use in the perspective of social disorganization are generally immersed in the large research literature of deviance, crime, and social problems. There are focused inquires on drug dealing, drink problems, and substance abuse in perceivably disorganized communities, such as Indian reservation camps in isolated regions and ethnic minority neighborhoods throughout major metropolitan areas (Sutter 1972; Higgins, Albrecht, and Albrecht 1977; Jensen, Stauss, and Harris 1977; Venkatesh 1996; Ennett, Flewelling, Lindrooth, and Norton 1997; Bourgois 1998a, 1998b; Mazerolle, Kadleck, and Roehl 1998; Scheier, Botvin, and Miller 1999; Johnson, Larson, Li, and Jang 2000). But an enduring research tradition has yet to be formed through systematic theorizing and multiple empirical explorations.

THEORETICAL FRAMEWORK

The social disorganization perspective looks into the social environment in which substance use occurs, fluctuates, persists, or desists. It focuses on how new or worsening physical conditions prompt moral decay or problems in value adjustment, paving the way for substance use and deviant behavior.

Definition

Social disorganization is a state of physical deterioration, spiritual disorientation, and general disorder or chaos in a society. Reflected in the experience of individuals, it is a period of stress, loss of control, pain, and suffering.

Social disorganization takes place when a society undergoes fundamental change in a short period of time. Reform, revolution, industrialization, urbanization, and modernization are usual forces leading to social disorganization. Job transfer, family relocation, migration, and immigration are typical causes of individual fear, frustration, and misadjustment.

There are two major dimensions in which social disorganization manifests itself. In the material dimension, it includes massive or constant migration, urban slums, rural desertion, erosion, dilapidated housing, unfinished and ongoing construction, unregulated traffic, noise, graffiti, and streets strewn with litter and trash. In the nonmaterial dimension, social disorganization invokes panic, restlessness, overblown optimism, ill-perceived opportunism, moral confusion, cynicism, loss of hope, depression, and mental illness. The two dimensions reinforce each other as people in despair find no support from their disorderly and alienating environment.

As far as substance use is concerned, social disorganization provides conditions for substance use to start and continue. However, as it exacerbates, substance use may feed back on social disorganization, making it more explicit, severe, or long-lasting in a particular environment.

Theoretical Image

People move from place to place. Society changes from time to time. When people leave their familiar environment and plunge into a new situation, they are homesick, long for their old ways of life, resist change or adjustment, and suffer from culture or location shock. When society switches from one structure, mode of operation, or type of solidarity to another, people and institutions are thrown out of balance and order. People struggle in confusion, helplessness, and pain. Old institutions break down. New institutions are yet to be established. As social change takes place constantly throughout history and across the globe, social disorganization becomes a universal phenomenon in human life.

Substance follows social disorganization as an evil, godmother, or accomplice. As an evil, substance lures dislocated people into drunkenness, abuse, addiction, dependency, or mental illness. It fills disorganized neighborhoods with traffic accidents, drug-dealing activities, prostitution, gang battles, uncleaned needles and syringes, cigarette butts, noises and sirens, or mourning for the dead. As a godmother, substance promises losers, sufferers, drug addicts, and other desperate people hopes for success, relief from pain, or treatments toward recovery. It attracts attention and investment into the community from mass media, policymakers, media professionals, and service personnel. As an accomplice, substance joins sojourners or their left-behind loved ones in their loneliness, despair, or suffering. It falls upon troubled families and communities with increasing levels of quarrels, traumatic events, drug traffic, police patrolling, and service intervention. Stress intensifies. The quality of life declines. Physical conditions worsen. Social disorganization therefore spreads and persists.

Substance use is a reaction to and a syndrome of social disorganization. Migrants and newcomers frequent bars, dancing clubs, and other substance-serving facilities because they are away from their families, they are lonely, and they are frustrated in search of jobs, opportunities, and economic fortunes from place to place. Family members left behind by migrants and emigrants engage in substance use because they are worried, they are bored, and they long for the safe return of their loved ones. In a disorganized family or neighborhood, people turn to drug dealing and sales for a living because they are not able to see any other effective means of survival in their environment. People spend welfare checks, drug profits, and other legal or illegal gains on substances because they do not have any tangible reference from which they learn to save for buying a house, renting a clean apartment, going to school, receiving vocational training, or acquiring some useful possessions. People smoke cigarettes, drink alcohol, or use drugs because they are idle, they are aimless, and they are entrenched in their familial, tribal, ethnic, or territorial enclave. Taking any disorganized social unit as a whole, substance use figures in almost inevitably and universally, along with crime, deviance, and other problems, as part of its general disorganization syndrome.

Substance users are social voices, representatives, or witnesses of disorganized families, neighborhoods, communities, and societies. Disorganization, as it takes place within some isolated social units or as it is experienced by some individuals, is not always obviously noticeable to other individuals, other social units, the whole population, or the mainstream society. It becomes known to the outside or the general public only when people going through or suffering from it speak out. Substance users qualify as representative voices of social disorganization because they are prompted into substance use often by their unique and salient experience with a disorganized environment. They serve to embody or epitomize social disorganization because they expand, diversify, or intensify their social disorganization experience through substance use. Even after they leave behind their disorganized nightmares and are able to incorporate substance intake into their regular life routine, they may still act as living witnesses of past incidence of disorganization within themselves or between them and their environment. Only through their vivid life stories can the truth be revealed as to how substance use makes its onset, escalates, tapers off, or ceases in the folding and unfolding of individual, group, organizational, communal, and social disorganization.

Over time, substance use increases in periods, generations, or eras of depression, epidemic, turmoil, war, reform, revolution, transition, and other traumatic events or dramatic changes. It decreases when people settle into their new lifestyle and society stabilizes in its new order. In the contemporary era, although some developed countries enjoy relatively long political stability, economic prosperity, and cultural consistency, substance use still remains high among citizens of those nations. The situation points to the existence of relative deprivation, regional disorganization, and cultural disenfranchisement in an overall organized social environment. Another possibility is: wealth corrupts morality and affluence promotes indulgence. People spoiled by material abundance fall into the same void of moral regulation as those who are forced into poverty, pain, and distress.

Across the globe, substance use skyrockets in countries that undergo transformations from civil war to national construction, from dictatorship to democracy, from tradition to modernity, from isolation to integration, from purism to pluralism, from controlled to market economies, and from poverty to development. Following soldiers, migrants, and emigrants, substance use remains prevalent and high in barracks, guerilla camps, transportation hub and corridor cities, slums, ethnic enclaves, transient lodges, train and bus stations, and other sojourner gathering places. Between poor and rich, developing and developed countries, the former prey on the latter's materialistically spoiled and morally decaying citizens, supplying tons of marijuana, heroin, cocaine, and other controlled substances through various underground channels. The latter prey on the former's often curious, innocent, and unsophisticated youth, women, and middle-class professionals as well as struggling underclass, dumping loads of alcohol, coffee, cigarettes, fragrances, synthetic foods and beverages, pharmaceutical products, and other consumer goods in the name of trade, emergency assistance, and economic aid. Crossing national borders, substance and substance use become part of social disorganization and reorganization in the world dynamics.

Theoretical Components

Conceptualized generally as a state of normlessness, loss of control, and disorder in the process as well as in the aftermath of change, disorganization can be systematically examined in six major components with respect to substance use and abuse.

Cause: Level of Change

Change is the primary cause of social disorganization. Although inquiry is made into sudden, dramatic change in a short span of time by sociologists, there is a general lack of attention to other modes of change by social disorganization researchers. In contemporary society, as change takes place constantly and instantly by way of scientific discovery and technological inventions, disorganization and reorganization can be part of ordinary life for any individual, organization, community, and even a whole country.

At the individual level, change may occur unilaterally, collaterally, or multilaterally, with or without interaction, in physical, psychological, interpersonal, and social dimensions. By natural law, one grows, matures, and ages from childhood, adolescence, and adulthood, to the senior stage. Adolescence, as a tumultuous period of time in life, usually features initiation, experimentation, and problematic experience in substance use. The senior stage, accompanied by social isolation and poor health, may witness increasing dependence on substance, including prescription drugs. In interaction with the environment, one may contract disease, inflict injury upon his or her body, develop fear or idiosyncrasy, or acquire certain medical conditions. To correct or sustain some of his or her normal or abnormal conditions, one may lock him- or herself up into an enduring relationship with substance. On the social front, one may move from marriage to divorce, employment to joblessness, high status to low position, affluence to poverty, or generally from success to failure. Caught in unfavorable change, one may turn to substance use as a coping strategy and mechanism.

Change at the social level involves family, group, organization, community, culture, or the entire society. There are first changes in collective attitudes, feelings, and sentiments. A prosubstance attitude by parents, organizational stakeholders, community leaders, and celebrities may fuel interest by children, employees, residents, and the general public in substance and substance use. There are then changes in law, rule, regulation, way of conducting business, standards, and morality. Prohibition and war on drugs deter the populace from drug dealing and use. They may also be responsible for the hardening of drug policy critics, drug legalization arguments, drug sales in inner-city neighborhoods, and drug abuse among socially depressed populations. There are finally changes in the structure and practice of social groups. For example, opening a coffee shop on the first floor of a high-rise office building may promote coffee consumption among people who work in the building. Bulldozing a few drug-infested city blocks for a community park by the municipal authority may eliminate drug and its related problems from the neighborhood. Providing vocational training for disadvantaged residents and expanding job opportunities to impoverished communities may reduce drug dealing and use in a whole city.

Cause: Form of Change

Among various changes leading to social disorganization, three major forms are most common. One is migration. People voluntarily or involuntarily leave their familiar lifestyle and daily routine for a new environment when they search for economic fortunes, take up new enterprises, or forge new personal relationships. Migrants generally divide into two groups. One group includes adventurers, explorers, critics, or rebels who are not satisfied with their existing conditions and want to explore new opportunities in an alien environment. They are confident about their own capabilities and usually have high expectations for themselves. However, when they fail in their endeavors, especially in a repeated or surprising fashion, they can fall into total despair and depression. Substance and substance use may then become their tools to vent anger, cope with stress, or punish themselves. Substance and substance use may even become their ultimate retreat from active social life. The other group consists of people who are forced out of employment, marriage, or family, or transferred from one school, one job assignment, or one foster care environment to another. They do not embrace the new environment and can become upset merely by the change they have to face in their life. For example, farmers drink to express their sorrow as well as boost their courage when they reluctantly leave their marginalized rural community for an unknown life in the city.

Another form of change is immigration. Immigrants leave their home society to enter a new country when they obtain a job, attend school, fulfill personal responsibility, or escape from war, poverty, or persecution. In an increasingly globalizing world, it is typical that people from developing societies pursue higher education in advanced countries, people from impoverished nations seek manual labor in affluent societies, and people from developed economies work on aid, technical, and investment projects in undeveloped regions. Compared to migration within a country, immigration across national borders involves language barriers, cultural clashes, national conflicts, and other system-level differences. Immigrants may long be cut off from their family due to travel and communications restrictions one country imposes upon the citizens of another. When a family gets together on foreign land, it may not be able to stay together at all because members are already forced apart in their individual lifestyle. Substance and substance use can come as a natural companion and automatic choice when immigrants, as they so often do, suffer from personal loneliness, family collapse, job discrimination, economic deprivation, and social mistreatment in a territory where they are identified as aliens.

Still another form of change is environmental. In the contemporary era, science and technology continuously push people into the frontier, exposing them to new knowledge, new information, and new ways of life. Mass media bring people instant news and reports, keeping them abreast of events and developments across the globe. Advanced communication and transportation networks move people from place to place, pushing them away from individual statics into overall social dynamics. Across the political landscape, officials are voted in and out. Policy changes when one party replaces the other to take control of government. In the economic arena, production, employment, and consumer confidence go up and down. The stock market rallies in response to good news and upbeat projections. It tumbles and even crashes when bad news converges from various sectors or the whole economic system. In fashion and culture, one style, vogue, ideology, or trend rises and dominates while the other declines and decays. Celebrities are born and buried. Books are read and abandoned. Amid all these changes, there are actors, witnesses, and the general reacting public. Although the main actors, such as politicians, investors, entrepreneurs, social activists, and celebrities, bear the greatest impact of change, the general public also feels the effects of a changing cycle. Most important, ordinary people, who form the mass of social dynamics, are the ultimate creators, enforcers, and sufferers of constant and instant change. The prevalence and salience of change in contemporary life may therefore serve as a general background or bottom line for substance use, abuse, and dependency across modern and postmodern society.

Manifestations: Material Dimension

Disorganization manifests in both material and nonmaterial dimensions. The material dimension concerns physical health, family situation, neighborhood condition, and overall social background. Society going through disorganization is likely to see overcrowded transportation hubs and lines, abandoned villages or towns, slums, deserted city districts, economic volatility, political instability, and even war. A community impacted by disorganization is likely to bear graffiti, litter, noise, dilapidated housing, violence, gang fighting, and a high flow of people into and out of its territory. A family experiencing disorganization may witness idled family plots, unattended yards, suffocating smells in the house, unwashed dishes, uncleaned beds and closets, as well as heightened hostility and tension among members. Individuals suffering from disorganization may look dirty and smell bad. They may move restlessly and aimlessly from place to place. They may complain about discomfort, pain, and some strange ailments. Beaten down by disorganization, they are indeed highly vulnerable for a variety of infections and diseases.

Physical conditions in association with disorganization may prompt, support, sustain, or exacerbate substance use. Individuals in pain are likely to seek relief from substance. Family members in dispute may find alcohol a perfect weapon to express their dissatisfaction, resentment, and rebellion. They do not seem to care much if they mess up things when they become drunk, as the house is already so often in disarray. Unlighted street corners, dirty public restrooms, and throngs of beggars, homeless people, and sojourners in train stations, bus depots, and downtown skid rows tend to attract and hide smoking, drug dealing, and substance use. So do shabby apartments, trash-strewn streets, and neon-lighted bars, dancing halls, or liquor stores. International drug traffickers target countries in civil war, of a corrupt or frequently changing government, or with a struggling economy. They also take advantage of ports and border regions involving multiple jurisdictions and huge flows of exports and imports. As they grow, manufacture, and transport substances in and through those disorganized countries and regions, they also create and sustain a substance use-and-abuse scene in local societies.

Manifestations: Spiritual Dimension

The nonmaterial or spiritual dimension of social disorganization concerns national ideology, public mentality, community sentiment, family unity, and individual morality. Under social disorganization, individuals are caught between their familiar habits, attitudes, and feelings and a not-so-familiar environment. They are shocked when they see people become rich or poor overnight, as they believe so deeply in hard work, honesty, justice, fairness, and progressive success. They feel uncomfortable, shamed, or offended when they face questions or are given warnings by the police regarding a party featuring some of their favorite substances, because they used to feel free to have a lot of fun and laughter at such gatherings with friends and relatives in their home countries or communities. Out of frustration or in hopelessness, spiritually disorganized individuals may turn to substances to drown care in the wine bowl, to develop some illusion about reality, or just to make a trip to a fantasized wonderland.

Families torn apart by social disorganization struggle between tradition and adventure, marriage and separation, status quo and opportunity, or persistence and change. One side fails in adaptation to reality while the other bears guilt for abandoning the family heritage. Socialization of children becomes problematic. The new generation grows up with the same level of ambivalence experienced by the old generation. Contradiction in beliefs, values, and social norms first confuses family members in their attitudes toward substance and substance use, making them easy prey of either pro- or antisubstance elements in their environment. It may also predispose some family members to substance abuse and dependency as they take blame, look for escape, or wrestle with moral dilemma.

In a disorganized community, people are either bitterly divided on moral standards or in a general state of cynicism, disorientation, or anomie. There are no agreed-upon spiritual inspirations, role models, and successful routes. John is tough and survives well in the neighborhood. But he is pursued by the police. Jennifer is different and works hard toward a professional career out of the community. But she looks so unique in her life endeavor that nobody else in the community feels even close to emulating her. In fact, her success story only serves to convince the others that this is where they deserve and belong. Settling into their communal environment, some residents drink alcohol to deal with idleness, some pick up unfinished cigarettes in the street and finish one after another, some cash in their welfare check for a binge, some trade their flesh for a "fix," and the majority remain just indifferent in their day-to-day journey through every extreme of life.

In the larger context, a culture, society, or country stricken by social disorganization is likely to fall into a vacuum or under a poverty of moral guidance, legal restraint, national unity, and political leadership. People rise to power, theory gains currency, and wealth develops into dominance, beyond conventional apprehension. Property dissipates into naught, fashion loses luster, and people fall in disgrace, out of commonsensical reasoning. There is a phenomenal lack of sharing in public concerns, collective sentiments, national ideology, and cultural symbols. People feel anything goes but nothing holds. Social attitudes toward substance and substance use therefore become divided. Public policies swing between liberalism, legalization, or promotion and conservatism, prohibition, or suppression. Drug dealers move in, following the loopholes created by prohibition or a tolerant climate brought by liberalism. Substance users are hounded unpredictably by prevention, treatment, rehabilitation, encouragement, condemnation, or punishment. The general scene in substance and substance use can go wildly up and down or remain constantly high as social disorganization rages on.

Outcome: System Disequilibrium and Demise

Social disorganization breaks out in a definable time span. It may push a system to the brink of collapse or put it into demise. It may take a system to reorganization and rebirth. It may also perpetuate its characteristic conditions for a system, placing it in institutionalized disorganization.

Individuals attacked by social disorganization may commit suicide. They may die involuntarily after traumatic experiences, such as physical exhaustion, mental breakdown, pain, suffocation, alcohol poisoning, and drug toxication. They may develop an enduring lifestyle to fit themselves into their disorganized environment. They may acquire a recurring mental condition to disable themselves from normal social functioning. For example, they live in slums, becoming receptive to poverty, violence, and crime in their surroundings. They drink heavily and continuously, taking alcohol as their main interest in life. They shoot drugs, befriending prostitutes, needle and syringe suppliers, and drug dealers. They engage in drug dealing and criminal offense, taking up a career in the nonconventional world. They are indifferent to their appearance, physical health, and the cleanliness of their immediate environment. They wander in the street, day by day, without any motivation for productive activity.

They are now passive, now active, now happy, now sad, roller-coastering from one extreme to the other. Addiction, drug dependency, criminal career, emotional instability, mental illness, and an unproductive lifestyle as a whole each epitomizes an individually habitualized response to social disorganization.

Groups, organizations, and communities rampaged by social disorganization may break down, be deserted, remain in ruins, or vanish from existence. They may also survive as its sites when social disorganization becomes institutionalized. Bearing social disorganization on a long-term basis, groups struggle with ever-changing membership, leadership, philosophy, and activity. Organizations scramble for direction amid conflicting ideals, goals, management styles, rules, and regulations. Communities hold their ground with difficulty as people move around, materials flow in and out, and social problems strike here, there, and everywhere. Group unity, organizational coherence, and community solidarity are low. Uncertainty, insecurity, and fear are widespread. Substance makes its constant onslaught as there is no agreed-upon attitude toward substance, there is barely coordinated action against substance use, and people find substance and substance use an easy way to avoid or deal with life in their disorganized environment.

Cultures, societies, and countries tortured by social disorganization may fall, collapse, and become extinct. They may also carry on as disorganized entities featuring year-old feuds among major social elements or general strife across the whole system. Productivity remains low since energy, intelligence, and wealth are buried in fear, suspicion, hatred, and fighting. Society is held back because it is divided and undecided about what is right, righteous, and rightful. Substance is used to distract attention, dispel fear, defuse stress, cure wounds, kill pain, boost morale, fuel hatred, or flare tension. Substance use becomes sanctified, professionalized, institutionalized, mystified, marginalized, or demonized. Substance users differentiate as warriors, heroes, deserters, traitors, losers, victims, or enemies. In a historically disorganized society, for instance, one ethnic group may honor a substance while the other ethnic group in conflict prohibits it as a taboo.

Outcome: Reorganization

Reorganization following disorganization provides a classical example of negative turning into positive. After a period of difficult struggle, individuals emerge in confidence, assertiveness, and balance. They speak the local language, engage in local business, participate in local activities, network with local residents, and begin to perceive themselves as part of the community, culture, and social environment in which they live. Their past experience no longer exists as a burden or an obstacle to new adventures. The relationship they maintain with old friends no longer prevents them from exploring the social mosaic of their new surroundings. In fact, as they are able to keep the past in proper perspective with the present and the future, they benefit from their past experience and former friendships as sources of inspiration, encouragement, and support. As far as substance and substance use are concerned, they definitely leave behind the time of heavy, uncontrollable, or self-hurting use when they are stricken most by social disorganization. In their reborn life, they either stay abstinent from substance or use substance in a way that is only congruent to their new environment.

A reorganized group, organization, or neighborhood appears not only in a new physical outlook, but also with a fresh collective spirit. Infighting ceases. Consensus develops. Leadership holds. Offices, streets, and gathering places are neat and clean. Police patrol in the community. Security guards stay on duty in various positions. Production, business, and other activities proceed in an orderly manner. On the spiritual level, members of the collective place trust in one another. They keep an eye on one another's kids, property, and belongings. They remain ready to offer help, to seek assistance, or to come together for emergency situations. Some residents may even join in volunteer teams to clean the streets, to keep order, to care for the needy, or to just stay alert for crime, drug dealing, gang activity, and other social problems that almost ruined their community in the near past. Substance is regulated. Substance dealing is kept out of the community. Substance use is put in check. Substance users are given medical treatment, emotional support, and life-related assistance. The whole community remain informed and educated about all the ramifications, legal, moral, health, and personal, of substance and substance use in their particular communal climate.

A new culture, society, or country may come into being in the aftermath of social disorganization. The reborn culture can be a combination of tradition and modernity, conservatism and liberalism, or ethnocentrism and cosmopolitanism. The positive of both sides is lightened while the negative is dimmed. In the political arena, the family, tribe, or elite-based authoritarian regime recedes from power, giving rise to democracy and pluralism. The economy changes from underdevelopment to development, from state planning to market rationality, and from self-sufficiency to global participation. The general population becomes educated, informed, open-minded, and future-oriented. The whole society or country stands firm and strong as a diversified, rejuvenated, and balanced system. On the matter of substance and substance use, laws, rules, and regulations are reasonably set up so that people can freely enjoy nutritional, medical, and recreational benefits of all different substances while seriously taking responsibility for their harmful consequences. Information is made widely available. Support is provided by both private and public sources. There is no crusade, blame, shaming, and criminalization against substance users, but only advice, warning, treatment, and support for them. Use and social reaction to substance overall remain slow, steady, and stable, in proper perspective with various important issues in life and on social agenda.

Theoretical Applications

The social disorganization perspective connects substance, substance use, and substance users to the general social environment and its change. A wide range of questions arise for theoretical exploration under this perspective.

First is the chain of reaction from change to substance use. The normally recognized or suspected sequence is that environment changes suddenly, individuals fall into maladaptation or misadjustment, normative control loosens while physical conditions deteriorate, and substance use begins or increases as people struggle in fear, uncertainty, and pain. Following the supposed sequence, what makes the environment or social structure change suddenly and drastically—industrialization, urbanization, economic reform, change of government, war, cultural revolution, natural disasters, or epidemics? Among people who are thrown into the process of change, what percentage lead, embrace, bear, or run away from the change? Are those who merely bear the change more vulnerable to maladaptation and misadjustment? Why does normative control loosen? Is it due to the fact that conflicting values, beliefs, and ideologies run rampant in the changing social environment? Is it because individuals are at a loss between their old and new environments? Why do physical conditions deteriorate? Are social assets destroyed? Are social resources redistributed, leaving some areas in severe depravation and poverty? Most important, how does moral decline combine with physical deterioration to conceive, support, and sustain substance use? What positive or negative functions does substance use serve for people in despair as well as communities in disorganization? Is substance use a mere symptom of social organization? Is it an integral part of social disorganization? Or is it an added factor that makes social organization more revealing?

Second is the proportional contribution of change in the environment versus change in personal actions. Change in the environment, such as economic development, market crash, and policy shift, occurs beyond individual control. Change in personal actions, such as relocation, taking a new job, and reuniting with the family, takes place out of individual choice. There are, however, interactions between environmentally originated and individually initiated changes. Environmental change triggers adaptive change by individuals whereas individual change may push one into a new environment or a new perception of the existing environment. Questions springing up then include: is environmental change more devastating in its consequence? If it impacted the general population, would it lead to widespread misadjustment, substance use, and deviance? Would the fact that everyone feels the pain and strain of change provide people with some collective buffer against social disorganization? In the case of individual change, is it less drastic and destructive in its effect? Since it only changes the social experience for particular individuals, would it correspondingly only result in isolated incidences of deviance or substance abuse? Would the fact that only one individual experiences the change alienate him or her in some relative deprivations? On the more delicate and complex side, how much can substance use and other disorganization-related problems be blamed on individual unwillingness or inability to adapt in the event of a large-scale uprooting social change? How much influence for individual deviations, including substance abuse and criminal behavior, can be traced to the lack of support or discriminatory practice from the environment when individuals undergo drastic change in their work and personal life?

Third is the inconstancy of change in contrast to the habituation of substance use. Change is constant in terms of social progress and individual maturation. It is inconstant in terms of personal disruption and social disorganization. Change comes and goes. Society alternates between stability and instability. Individuals experience turbulence amid peace and peace amid turbulence. On the other hand, substance is addictive, substance use is habitual, and substance users can become lifelong addicts. One might ask: Would disorganization-prompted substance use come and go in response to disorganization itself? If substance use remains as a habit, an addictive state, or a disease, would users be less or more prepared for yet another possible round of social disorganization breaking out in their environment or exploding from their personal life? If substance use rises and recedes along with disorganization, can it be legitimately called disorganization-specific or characteristic use, different from any other use caused by or taking place in nondisorganization situations?

Finally, questions can be identified and explored between substance use and social reorganization. For instance, would substance use be institutionalized as an integral part of new social order when most users pick it up as a habit in the time of social disorganization? Would it have to be first demonized and eliminated before any social reorganization could begin because it lies so deeply in the core of all evils of social disorganization?

Empirical Tests

The social disorganization perspective touches upon both the statics and dynamics of target research issues as it relates them to social change in the larger environment. It creates a prime opportunity to apply, expand, and enrich different research methods in the study of substance use and abuse.

Case studies are indispensable to following individuals who plunge into a new environment because of job transfer, marriage, family reunion, imprisonment, or exile, or due to relocation, migration, or immigration. Studies can be conducted to see how a new worker, a new inmate, or a newcomer attempts to fit into his or her environment, what hardship he or she has to bear, what compromise he or she has to make, and how he or she resists or turns to substance in the process of resettlement. Face-to-face interviews can be arranged to allow research subjects to reveal their most inner feelings and subtlest adjustment in the process of change. Personal documents, including diaries, letters, and medical records, may also be analyzed to shed light on the general process an individual has to go through, from excitement, suspicion, hostility, rejection, and accommodation, to acceptance, in his or her new environment. Approaching substance use and abuse as legal, moral, and character-implicating issues, researchers may make an effort to cultivate emotional rapport with their research subjects so that they can gain access to rare occasions or materials and gather information about secret coping strategies through personal trust.

Historical analysis is suitable to study major social transformations in a culture or territory. Scholarly publications, media presentations, public records, official statistics, novels and other fiction, and folk literature can be collected and analyzed to develop a general picture of social disorganization in the time of religious reform, cultural renaissance, economic development, or political realignment. For example, the number of migrants or immigrants on governmental records may be indicative of the level of social mobility or instability. Sales volume in alcohol, tobacco, and other licit substances from commercial sources may reveal the prevalence of substance consumption. Interdiction and confiscation figures on controlled substances by custom, coast guard, and law enforcement may present a bottom line for illicit drug dealing, possession, and use. Relating key variables and their appropriate indicators to one another, researchers can identify and explore correlations and even some causal relationships about critical events taking place in a particular historical era.

Survey research is a timely device to document social change in the making. In the enormously diverse and rapidly changing world, researchers can study almost all possible social disorganization scenes, from war, genocide, terrorism, industrialization, urbanization, technological innovation, cultural or ethnic marginalization, migration, immigration, epidemics, natural disasters, and job relocation, to divorce. A representative or nonrepresentative sample of respondents can be selected from the population or a segment of the population who undergo a specific social disorganization experience. Questions can be asked about their collective as well as individual encounters with disruptive social change. Does substance figure in their reaction to social disorganization, and how? For example, in refugee camps, refugees running away from war, natural disasters, economic hardship, or political persecution can be studied through face-to-face interview or self-administered survey to see if substance use is reduced, contained, increased, or worsened when they are not only cut off from their old environment, but also restricted from assimilating into their new society. Most important, constant monitoring of contemporaries through regular opinion polls and ad hoc research surveys can provide critical insights about substance use, social change, and their interactions across a culture, a country, a region, and even the whole world.

Experimental studies can be used to ascertain the causal effect of social disorganization on substance use and abuse. In quasi-experimental designs, individuals, families, organizations, neighborhoods, cultures, countries, or historical periods are identified in comparable groups to see if social disorganization causes and accounts for the difference in substance use and other deviations when major characteristic variables pertaining to the compared groups remain constant or identical. For instance, two societies are selected for comparison when they are similar in key aspects, such as population composition, culture, and political system, and differ only in social disorganization experience: one switches from state planning to a market economy while the other stays on its original economic course. If an increase in substance use is found in one society but not the other, the change may then be legitimately attributed to the widespread breakdown of public enterprises, massive unemployment, and the difficult rise of market-driven business endeavors in the process of economic reform. Beyond naturally occurring events, some experimental conditions can be man-made to examine various effects of social disorganization, especially how normative contradiction or a lack of normative control affects people and their behavior. Between two otherwise similar groups, for example, one is given intensive educational sessions in which their core values are questioned, ridiculed, and attacked while the other is allowed to continue their normal way of thinking and acting. A wealth of information about moral confusion, normative void, and their respective behavioral reaction, including substance use, can be gathered if the two groups are properly controlled within the time frame as well as the spatial boundary of the experimental design.

POLICY IMPLICATIONS

The social disorganization perspective places substance users in their changing social environment. The contextual, systematic, and dynamic approach it takes in theoretical analysis can have profound implications and impacts for policy and social actions toward substance and substance use.

Public Health

In the spirit of the social disorganization perspective, public health officials and professionals react to substance use as an epidemic, not as individual acts. To prevent substance use, they make efforts to educate the general public about the changing social environment and a health lifestyle in response to change, both constant, gradual and accidental, sudden. They engage in scientific research for systematic knowledge about social change, stress, mental illness, health hazards, substance use, and their interrelations. They provide specific advice and counseling on how to deal with change and how to avoid or regulate substance use in the time of turmoil and difficulty. They reach out to troubled neighborhoods, such as downtown skid row areas, ethnic enclaves, and refugee camps. They target vulnerable populations, such as immigrants, vagrants, homeless people, and migrant prostitutes. By providing immunizations, delivering condoms, exchanging needles and syringes, and offering other health services, they may prevent isolated risks and incidents from breaking out into large-scale epidemics.

To intervene in substance use, health officials and professionals customize treatment in congruence with the cultural, ethnic, and emotional needs of their clients and patients, and deliver it directly to the family, group, or community impacted by social disorganization. They not only treat symptoms of substance use, but also address moral and emotional conditions that prompt and sustain substance use. They not only treat individual users, but also organize them into self-help groups. For instance, clients and patients are encouraged to describe their shared social disorganization experience and suggest collectively effective solutions for their substance use and other social problems. Health officials and professionals set up service stations in areas where social disorganization–impacted populations are concentrated. They even follow clients and patients from street to street, and from neighborhood to neighborhood. To ensure clients and patients persist in recovery from substance dependency, they work with educational institutions, vocational training centers, businesses, and government agencies to integrate medical treatment with social support in comprehensive packages.

Social Control

Social control agencies and agents can benefit from the social disorganization perspective by changing their focus from individual to community, from intervention to prevention, and from coercive control to social support. Instead of targeting particular individuals, they can map out the whole territory under jurisdiction and increase their presence in the most problematic areas. In target areas, they can set up local stations. They may increase patrolling frequency and intensity. Patrolling officers may switch from automobile to bicycle and foot patrols. They may practice community policing to connect to local residents and businesses, and to combine control with service.

On the physical level, control agencies and agents introduce laws or ordinances to regulate and restrict the presence of tobacco billboard advertisements, the volume of alcohol sales and consumption, and the distribution of adult entertainment in the neighborhood. They work with local businesses and residents to clean the street, to remove graffiti, and to keep stores and houses in decent shape. Local authorities and services make sure that streets are properly lighted, trash is collected on schedule, and parks are supplied with adequate amenities. Drug dealers are chased from the community. Substance users are referred to appropriate locations for treatment and assistance.

Spiritually, laws are made and enforced so that immigrants and other types of newcomers are not discriminated against on the job, or in business, service, and welfare agencies, as well as in social contact. Politicians speak out for social equity, fairness, and openness. Community leaders agitate for compassion and mutual support. Mass media educate people about social change and strategies for dealing with change. Religious and nonprofit organizations render tangible assistance to people in need. Volunteers deliver printed brochures and oral messages in ethnic languages or local dialects. Law enforcement agencies and agents serve as public models and examples for the sanctity of law, authority, and social order. Nobody feels left out or behind on important social issues, including the legality of substance and the harm or benefit of substance use, as the whole community or society remains cohesively as an informed collective.

Life and Community

Community bears the impact of social disorganization. Community feels the strongest need to reorganize itself from a disorganized experience.

First, it is crucial that residents in the community develop a genuine interest in the long-term development of their proximate environment. In the time of social disorganization, people flock into a neighborhood. They take refuge in the neighborhood. They consider it only a pathway toward their final destination. There is no feeling of home or sense of belonging. In fact, most residents believe and hope they will leave the community and settle in a better place. The prevailing sentiment of temporality among residents provides a soil for a general lack of concern for the community. Some beg money in the street or steal from local stores or apartments because they feel they can leave anytime. Some litter the public areas or walk around in drunkenness because they see everyone doing the same.

Outsiders also tend to take advantage of the known transience of the community. They regularly or irregularly invade the community with drug dealing, robbery, violence, and other criminal activities. The community therefore is exploited both from within and from without. A cultivation of identification with the neighborhood is obviously key to breaking the negative cycle for positive community renewal.

Second, it is critical that residents in the community build mutual support among themselves. Social disorganization can throw people into tension and distrust. People may curse, cheat, rob, or fight one another when they are forced to compete for limited resources, expose their privacy, or live in relative deprivation. For example, some residents automatically suspect their neighbors of theft and other offenses because they feel they are as desperate as themselves. Some intentionally or unintentionally sabotage their neighbors' efforts for positive change because they do not think the neighbors are more special than themselves and deserve something better. Businesses refuse to hire local people because they consider them junkies or thugs who either know too much about bad things or have too little impetus for good behavior. To reorganize the community, residents need to overcome their own stereotypes about themselves. Once they develop trust in themselves, they can then keep an eye on one another's children and property. They can form volunteer groups for neighborhood watch, street cleaning, and family counseling. Businesses extend help in charitable events and community activities. Messages about substances are spread in the neighborhood. Methods of abstinence or recovery from addiction are shared from individual to individual. The whole community thus turns into a network of support in which residents treat and draw upon each other as valuable resources.

Third, it is important that residents in the community open up to the outside world, welcoming newcomers and embracing positive interventions. Social disorganization falls upon individuals when they move from place to place. It worsens when people take refuge in their localized enclaves, refusing intervention from the outside. To assist newcomers, local residents can open their houses for temporary living, provide information about transportation, job opportunities, and life necessities, and share their experiences in various phases of life endeavors. Sometimes, a smile, a chat, a word of encouragement, an offer of help, a party, a picnic, or an excursion can make a newcomer feel welcomed and accepted into his or her new environment. For professional, legal, and governmental assistance from outside the community, residents need to understand that their community is part of the larger social environment. Treatment for and control of various social problems require resources and efforts beyond the community. For instance, dealing of controlled substances by organized crime groups warrants legally prescribed punitive action. Chemical dependency calls for medical attention. It is only through working with medical or social control authorities that people can effectively contain or eliminate those salient substance problems in their community.

Work and Organization

Work and organization are sources of social change and disorganization. They are also forces for social reorganization and stability.

From a social disorganization perspective, work and production are ultimate causes for technological innovation, economic development, political reform, and social progress. Work demands individual change in attitude and behavior. It requires transfer and relocation. It dictates migration, emigration, or immigration. While it cannot, nor should it, resist overall social change it creates with many other social institutions, an organization can and should assist its members in their individual adjustment to change. On the one hand, it can improve personnel policies, making promotion and demotion rational, predictable, and synchronized with individual career paths. It can rationalize production planning and configuration, avoiding and minimizing job reassignment and transfer. It can humanize relationships with labor, ensuring job security, providing on-job training and relearning opportunities, giving advanced notice in the unfortunate event of layoff, and assisting to-be-laid-off employees in their search for new jobs. On the other hand, an organization should give new recruits, transferred, reassigned, or demoted employees, as well as employees with language barriers and religious or ethnic complications appropriate breathing space in work assignment and job responsibility. Support can be offered in the form of vocation, gift, benefit, and bonus. Information may be made available through orientation, counseling, and brochure. By taking both preventive and corrective measures, an organization can obviously help its members reduce or eliminate their individual risk for social disorganization and its related deviations, including substance use and abuse.

Beyond its own membership, an organization itself is a member of the community. It serves as a basic reference for the community on a wide range of issues, such as openness to outsiders, fairness to newcomers, and nondiscriminative treatment of visitors or sojourners. The positive or negative approach taken by one individual business or organization can contagiously spread to others, giving a whole community a reputation as either a favorable or unfavorable place for newcomers, immigrants, or minorities. In the time of peace as well as during crisis, emergency, collective movement, or dramatic change, an organization can share its resources with the community. It can host regular open houses for local residents or open its facility as a public shelter in the aftermath of tragic incidents. It can make routine and emergency material and monetary contributions. It can offer local residents information, knowledge, and counseling on issues of its specialty or general interest. It can create jobs and extend work opportunities to members of the community. It may also send its employees to the community to clean the street and help people in need. In a community where businesses and organizations actively engage in various community affairs, not only are residents prepared for their individual social disorganization experience, but also the onslaught of any large-scale social disorganization is mitigated on the whole community. Substance use and other social problems can therefore be significantly prevented and reduced.

The social disorganization perspective explores the social environment and its critical change for answers and insights on substance use and abuse. Substance symbolizes a particular social context or historical era. Substance use reflects a specific reaction to social change or a peculiar feeling about life dynamics. Substance users are representatives of a population struggling against the strong current of change and movement in their social environment.

While environment is where people live, find support, and get used to, it is also what makes people feel alienated, discriminated against, and stressed out. While change is created, embraced, or chosen by people, it can also throw people into shock, despair, and maladjustment. Social disorganization occurs when people have difficulty dealing with change in life or have trouble adapting to their environment. In its spiritual dimension, social disorganization features a moral or normative vacuum. On the one hand, people find their old beliefs and values no longer serve their needs in the new environment. On the other hand, they feel it is difficult and even impossible to understand and acquire new norms. In the material manifestation, social disorganization is epitomized in physical disorderliness, mental illness, residential instability, neighborhood tension, urban decay, rising crime, widespread deviations, and other measurable social problems. Substance and substance use can figure in social disorganization in various ways, not only as individual coping mechanisms, but also as social by-products, not only as phenomenal symptoms, but also as substantive roots, not only as collateral consequences, but also as essential causes.

The social disorganization perspective highlights the importance of social forces and institutions versus individual choices and reactions in the study of substance use and abuse. It provides practical directions on how to prevent or reduce substance use and abuse in a changing social environment. It also gives realistic assessments of substance use and abuse over the dynamic process of human progress. In contemporary society, individuals are constantly bombarded with social and market changes fueled by scientific discoveries and technological innovations. The pace of life is demandingly fast. It can only become faster rather than slower when it moves further into the future. Substance use and abuse are certain to be prevalent and high as change and social disorganization become inevitable and salient elements in modern and postmodern life.

—8—

The Social Learning Perspective

Like climbing mountains, playing the piano, or growing crops, using substances is a human behavior. As human behavior, substance use takes place in certain contexts, follows particular cause-effect sequences, and involves specific efforts from mind and body, such as motivations, justifications, skills, and levels of performance.

The social learning perspective focuses on the behavioral dimension of substance use. It explores how substance use is acquired as a human behavior. Specifically, it studies what social situations are defined as favorable to, what motivations and rationalizations are required for, and what skills and techniques are involved in substance use. It also examines how the consequence of substance use feeds back on the process of learning and whether substance use can be unlearned through messages, groupings, and sources of influence unfavorable to violation of social norms.

SOURCES OF INSPIRATION

French social theorist Gabriel Tarde was one of the earliest scholars to formulate a learning perspective on deviance. Criticizing Durkheim's conception of society as a "thing in itself," Tarde (1912) drew attention to the social processes whereby ways of thinking and acting are passed on from group to group. Deviance, according to Tarde, originates and spreads as fads and fashions. People learn deviance through a social acquisition process governed by what he referred to as the "three laws of imitation." The three laws of imitation are: the law of close contact, the law of imitation of superiors by inferiors, and the law of insertion, which explains how power inherent in novelty assists in the replacement of old customs by new fashions (Tarde 1912).

The first systematic exposition of the social learning perspective, however, was provided by Edwin Sutherland. In *Principles of Criminology*, Sutherland (1934) hypothesized that "any person can be trained to adopt and follow" a pattern of criminal behavior (51). In *The Professional Thief*, Sutherland (1937) observed that "tutelage by professional thieves is essential for the development of skills, attitudes, codes, and connections, which are required in professional theft" (v–vi). The formal presentation of a theory of differential association appeared in the third edition of *Principles of Criminology* in 1939. But it was in the fourth edition of the textbook in 1947 that Sutherland offered a comprehensive explanation of criminal behavior by the theory of differential association. The theory consists of nine propositions: (a) criminal behavior is learned; (b) criminal behavior is learned in interaction with other persons in a process of communication; (c) the principal part of the learning of criminal behavior occurs within intimate personal groups; (d) when criminal behavior is learned, the learning includes both the techniques of committing the crime and the specific direction of motives, drives, rationalizations, and attitudes; (e) the specific direction of motives and drives is learned from definitions of the legal codes as favorable or unfavorable; (f) a person becomes delinquent because of an excess of definitions favorable to violation of law over definitions unfavorable to violation of law; (g) differential associations may vary in frequency, duration, priority, and intensity; (h) the process of learning criminal behavior by association with criminal and anticriminal patterns involves all of the mechanisms that are involved in any other learning; and (i) while criminal behavior is an expression of general needs and values, it is not explained by those general needs and values, since noncriminal behavior is an expression of the same needs and values (Sutherland 1947).

Is direct intimate contact with prodeviant people necessary for acquiring deviant behavior? People learn various ideas and acts indirectly by mass media and from distant reference groups. According to Daniel Glaser (1956), "a person pursues criminal behavior to the extent that he identifies himself with real or imaginary persons from whose perspective his criminal behavior seems acceptable" (440). In other words, differential identification, rather than differential association, is at the heart of deviant learning. People may never associate directly with some of their role models and reference groups. But as long as they identify with them, those role models and reference groups can essentially affect their definition of the world and further shape their actions within it.

Is there anything in the mainstream society deviants need to learn and deal with while specializing in language, morality, and norms of behavior appropriate for the deviant world? Deviants live in worlds of both conformity and nonconformity. To overcome the external constraints of conventional social control, they need to learn some rhetoric or vocabularies as their neutralizing techniques. To manage the internal feelings of shame, they need to learn some self-deceptive or manipulative methods as their protection strategies. For the former, Gresham Sykes and David Matza (1957) provide a list of five typical techniques: denial of responsibility, denial of injury, denial of victim, condemning the condemner, and appeal to higher loyalties. For the latter, Jack Douglas (1977) identifies such strategies as self-deception, self-seduction, aggressive countermoralism, and counterpride displays.

Is deviant learning governed by the principles of operant psychology? According to B. F. Skinner (1953), human behaviors are shaped by the consequences they produce. Some acts lead to positive, pleasurable, or desirable outcomes, such as the presence of rewards (positive reinforcement) or the removal of punishment (negative reinforcement). They are thus likely to be repeated in a similar fashion. Some acts result in negative, painful, or undesirable consequences, such as the presence of punishment (positive punishment) or the removal of rewards (negative punishment). They are thus not likely to be repeated in a similar fashion. Applying operant principles to the learning of criminal behavior, Robert Burgess and Ronald Akers (1966) reformulate Sutherland's theory of differential association in terms of a sequence of differentially reinforced and punished social experiences. Specifically, they develop the following major propositions in their theory of differential reinforcement: (a) deviant behavior is learned according to the principles of operant conditioning; (b) deviant behavior is learned in both social and nonsocial situations that are reinforcing for such behavior; (c) the learning of deviant behavior occurs in those groups that compose the individual's major source of reinforcements; (d) the learning of deviant behavior is a function of the available enforcers; (e) the probability that a person will commit deviant behavior changes with the discriminative value he has acquired over conforming behavior in the process of reinforcement; and (f) the strength of deviant behavior is a direct function of the amount, frequency, and probability of its reinforcement (Burgess and Akers, 1966; Akers 1977).

On substance use and abuse, Howard Becker's study of learning to become a marijuana smoker represents a classical application of the learning perspective. As Becker (1963) pointed out, new users learn marijuana smoking in association with good friends or positively perceived associates and through careful observation, imitation, and direct instruction. They first learn how to overcome any previous feelings about the immoral images of marijuana use. They then learn how to rationalize smoking as an acceptable behavior. For instance, they learn to believe that they can fake the appearance of normality while getting high, that they will not get caught, and that they will not become slaves to the drug. Finally, they learn how to cue into the proper techniques of smoking and to enjoy the physical effects of the drug in a pleasurable manner.

In practice, the learning perspective highlights the importance of association and social grouping to substance users and substance-related professionals, making reverse differential association and group unlearning major strategies for various self-help movements and treatment modalities. For instance, Alcoholics Anonymous encourages members to meet frequently and regularly in classes and at parties. They exchange testimonial admissions to being alcoholics, share personal stories of being "down and out," praise the wonders of Alcoholics Anonymous, and appreciate the benefits of the supportive understanding that only alcoholics care to provide for one another (Alcoholics Anonymous 1976). Synanon, a drug addiction rehabilitation organization, offers a nearly total learning environment for implementing the differential association perspective. Within it, participants are taught to hate drugs, suppress individual desires, and dissociate from deviant culture and former drug acquaintances. Learning is reinforced not only by continuous joint activities and family-style cohesion among members, but also by valuable social status granted for staying off drugs and developing antidrug attitudes (Volkman and Cressey 1963).

Recent developments from research and practice continue to show the influence of the learning perspective. In examining the learning of substance use through primary and secondary associations, some focus on sources of influence, from parents, to schoolmates, to co-workers (Sellers and Winfree 1990; Bell, Pavis, Cunningham-Burley, and Amos 1998; Donohew, Clayton, Skinner, and Colon 1999). Some compare different types of substances and different forms of use, from tobacco, to alcohol, to marijuana, to hard drugs (Corwyn, Benda, and Ballard 1997; Benda 1999; Epstein, Botvin, and Diaz 1999). Some look into the nature, strength, and change of associations. For example, Judy Andrews, Hyman Hops, and Susan Duncan (1997) analyzed data from 657 adolescents, 357 fathers, and 633 mothers over a six-year period. They found that all adolescents modeled mother's cigarette use and father's marijuana use, older adolescents modeled mother's marijuana use, and younger girls and older boys modeled father's alcohol use if they had a relatively good or moderate relationship with that parent, but did not model their parent's use if the relationship with that parent was relatively poor. Ronald Akers and Gang Lee (1999) traced the age-use curve in relation to social learning variables among 3,065 Midwestern adolescents in grades 7 to 12. They found that age variations in marijuana use are mediated by age-related variations in social learning, and to a lesser degree, that social bonding variables mediate the age–marijuana use relationship during adolescence.

In relating or applying learning principles to the prevention of substance use, some liken the process of cessation to that of initiation and the experience of abstinence to that of use (Winfree, Sellers, and Clason 1993; Akers and Lee 1996). Some follow group sessions and positive associations as prevention strategies and activities in different contexts, such as family, school, community, and employment organizations (Cook, Back, and Trudeau 1996; Capece and Akers 1995). Some explore the efficacy of innovative approaches in counteracting learned definitions favorable to violation of law and effecting positive attitudinal and behavioral changes among groups at risk for substance abuse (Gropper, Liraz, Portowicz, and Schindler 1995; Zack and Vogel-Sprott 1997). For example, an attractive, cartoon-illustrated computer program, when combined with games, role playing, and group techniques, may prove to be more effective in: (a) providing information about drugs and alcohol; (b) changing beliefs, attitudes, feelings, and values concerning drug and alcohol use; and (c) teaching drug-resistance, decision-making, and coping skills. However, for any excessive optimism toward the unlearning of substance use, Fin-Aage Esbensen and Delbert Elliott's (1994) event history analysis of eight waves of the National Youth Survey from 1976 to 1989 seems to offer a reality warning of caution. Based on data on drug use for 1,172 respondents aged 11 to 30, they find that once initiation has occurred, drug use is maintained for an extended time; demographic characteristics have very little effect on either initiation or resistance of drug use; variables representing social learning theory are more important in accounting for initiation than discontinuity of drug use; and life events, such as marriage and becoming a parent, increase the odds of discontinuing drug use.

THEORETICAL FRAMEWORK

The social learning perspective claims that substance use is a learned behavior. At the outset, it negates any essential influence from nature, in terms of either physical composition or mental properties. In the core of the theory, it explores form and content, cause and effect, subject and context, association and identification, morality and technicality, as well as structure and process of learning, in the acquisition of substance use as a human behavior.

Definition

Learning is a universal phenomenon in the animal world. Using their naturally born and developed senses, animals learn to communicate with one another within their own species, connect to organic and inorganic resources from their specific environment, and survive in nature against the odds of evolution and extinction. Human beings learn at the highest level, involving not only a higher level of intelligence, but also a complex system of language and symbols, culture and social norms, and theory and methods. Besides natural adaptations, human beings learn to understand the universe, change their existence, and create a world of their own.

Within human society, individuals learn to abide by a culture of practice, master a system of knowledge, assume a multitude of roles, and become the kind of persons they aspire to be.

The social learning perspective appreciates both the universality and the variety of learning within social groups, among human beings, and across the animal world. As a theory on crime and deviance, however, it focuses on why and how learning, specifically learning a socially disapproved behavior, still takes on a social outlook. First, learning is a group behavior. People learn things through interaction not isolation. Second, disapproval, like approval, is a social process. It involves the attribution of judgment by an established authority. Third, socially disapproved behavior earns its negative identification by actively challenging some mainstream practices. It is not just what is disallowed or prohibited but what triggers or activates current social reactions. Fourth, a socially distanced group maintains its marginal status by remaining in some part of the social scene. Its members are not forced into retreat from society but are constantly targeted by society as sources of threat, tension, and disorder.

Applied to substance use and substance users, the social learning perspective highlights: (a) substance use emerges at the confluence of various social forces existing in the contemporary era; (b) individuals learn to use substances at the confluence of various interpersonal influences they experience in their social environment; (c) substance use is transmitted from group to group, from place to place as people learn to justify use and build self-support amid social condemnation and attacks; (d) substance use is passed on from generation to generation, from time to time as people learn through primary associations, such as family and kinship, as well as secondary sources, such as the media and literature; and (e) use rationalizations, motives, and techniques proliferate while substance use expands and the number of substance users grows. An emerging subculture of substance use can provide an even more systematic and powerful learning environment for both novice and experienced learners to acquire and improve their thoughts and acts surrounding substance use.

Theoretical Image

Substance use is a learned behavior. Learning shapes the whole outlook as well as the major aspects of substances, substance use, substance users, substance use environments, and substance use evolution.

Beginning with substances, learning has been associated with the progress of human knowledge. In primitive societies and premodern times, people learned about a substance and its medicinal, nutritional, or psychedelic effects through trial and error. With advances in science and technology, people in the modern world have come to know a large inventory of medications, foods, and drugs in great detail. For each substance, they may analyze its chemical composition, identify which part of its molecule acts on what part of the human body, and synthesize the active agent in a series of similar substances. Natural substances are modified with artificial flavors. Synthetic drugs appear in natural forms. Consumers are pressured with various appeals and incentives to buy and use substances, from fine wine to freshly brewed beers, from handmade cigars to filtered cigarettes, and from health products to over-the-counter drugs. On illicit substances, while research and treatment have generated substantial knowledge about their respective chemical structure, neurobiological effects, use manifestations, and withdrawal symptoms, information has also been widely and effectively used in growing, processing, synthesizing, and preparing each of them for recreational consumption by people of different preferences, tastes, and socioeconomic status.

Substance use involves the learning of use motives, use justifications, methods of administration, and effect management. Although users learn things specific to their personal needs, substance of use, and situation of use, general knowledge and information are available for circulation and dissemination among users and across the public. For instance, use may be out of boredom, rebellion, or stress. Justifications can be made in terms of freedom of choice, possible benefits, or social pressure. Methods of administration include enteral and parenteral routes. By the enteral route, a substance is taken orally, sublingually, or rectally. In the parenteral route, drugs are administered through subcutaneous, intramuscular, or intravenous injections (Doweiko 1996). Finally, most substances have both primary and secondary effects. Effect management requires that users learn to enjoy primary while accommodating secondary effects.

Substance users vary in learning motivation, capability, and performance. Motivation concerns a user's motive, interest, and enthusiasm in experimenting with a new substance and its different methods of administration. A highly motivated user who actively seeks advice and information from various sources on a substance and its use differs from a user who naturally follows his or her parents in picking up a habit of use, and much more from a user who is forced into use by his or her close friends. Capability includes not only intellectual ability to perceive, understand, and master morality, knowledge, and techniques pertaining to substance use, but also physical capacity to accommodate the effects of a substance, to endure the symptoms of withdrawal, and to adapt to the habit of use. Some users may be quick to internalize user mentalities or to distinguish subtle effects from one method of use to another, while others may be slow in overcoming their initial reactions to a substance or justifying their use with a deeply felt pleasurable effect. Performance is a consequential variable of both motivation and ability. It measures the speed by which a user progresses from initiation to experimentation to habitual use, the frequency with which a user engages in use during a specific time period, and the intensity by which a user reacts to the presence and absence of a substance through specific routes and in specific amounts. For instance, some users learn to bear a higher level of intensity through injection, high dosage, or frequent administration, while others adjust to casual consumption by oral intake, dilution, or at-comfort exposure.

Substance use environments refer to both the macro social atmosphere in which substance use and users are perceived, evaluated, and treated, and micro associational groupings through which substance users learn and share ideas, motives, methods, skills, and other resources regarding substance use. Social atmosphere changes with science, technology, education, and mass media. Science provides empirical evidence about health effects of various substances, including alcohol, tobacco, and hard drugs. Education raises the level and scope of understanding about nature, human life, and health lifestyle. Technology and mass media spread knowledge and information, widely and pervasively, across the population. While social atmosphere follows all these learning-related domains, it determines how individuals learn and develop their attitudes and behaviors toward substance use. In contemporary society, as more and more people are educated about the hazardous consequences of alcohol and addictive substances to human health, more and more of them learn to avoid rather than to use those substances, even for recreational purposes. Similarly, associational groupings not only shape how substance users learn from one another, but also change as they create and exchange new vocabularies, techniques, and strategies in substance use. For instance, people usually learn to drink alcohol, smoke cigarettes, or use illicit drugs from family members, relatives, neighbors, classmates, or co-workers. Now with the emergence of a substance culture sustained by mass media, substance use is being contagiously transmitted from place to place through strangers, distant role models, age-related peers, or any aspects of human life, such as hairstyles, fashions, sexual orientation, homelessness, defects, or diseases. For instance, homeless people swallow one thing (their identifying substance) to stay vigilant in the darkness, homosexuals take another thing (their indicator drug) to maintain sexual functionality, and AIDS patients use still another thing (their marker substance) to manage pain and symptoms.

Finally, substance use evolution records how learning interacts with substance use over time. On the one hand, learning has gradually enlarged the inventory of substances known for human consumption as well as expanded the spectrum of use for each known substance. Compared to their ancestors hundreds of years ago, people in modern time have a far greater variety of substances, from natural to synthetic, from licit to illicit, and from name brand to generic, for a far greater variety of use, from nutrition to body enhancement, from disease prevention to health promotion, and from medical treatment to recreational entertainment. On the other hand, various substances available to use in different contexts for different purposes make learning more and more a horrendous task for individuals. Information spreads from one source to another, and changes from time to time. It is difficult to distinguish the valid from the invalid, the accurate from the inaccurate, and the credible from the incredible. There are manifest cases of overdose, intoxication, poisoning, drug interactions, side effects, loss of drug effects, and other forms of misuse or abuse. There are even more latent cases of unknown, unobservable, or inexplicable consequences by certain drugs to those who take the drugs due to misjudgment by learned professionals or misinformation available from allegedly learned sources. In other dimensions, the level, frequency, and intensity of substance use fluctuate with the scale of education and the depth of learning in societies across different times. While a larger inventory of substances known in modern time tends to make use and abuse more likely to occur, a better educated citizenry in open society has seemingly more rational reasoning to take a generally cautionary attitude toward all forms of substance use.

Theoretical Components

The social learning perspective explores various aspects of learning, from the foundation, modes, content, stages, and contingencies, to the social context of learning, in relation to substance use and users.

The Foundation of Learning: Nature versus Nurture

The learning perspective posits that substance use is learned through social interactions. Nurture, instead of nature, clearly and unequivocally constitutes the philosophical foundation of the learning perspective.

However, as an informed theory in contemporary time, the learning perspective does not negate the influence of nature. First, learning builds upon intelligence. Intelligence has been proved to be determined by not only postbirth development but also genetic composition. Users of higher intelligence may master use motives and techniques faster and more to the essence. Socially, they may rise to the higher echelon more easily and therefore have readier access to supply, better control of quality, and more refined support through subculture. Second, substance use relates to physical accommodation and tolerance. People with certain hereditary traits or bodily characteristics may possess a greater inclination to learn to use certain substances. Once they start, they not only learn fast but also tend to learn to be both intense and habitual users. For instance, some studies find alcoholism is inheritable from parents to children and further to grandchildren. Third, substance use, as a nurtured behavior, has direct consequences on the human mind and body, the product of nature. Some consequences can be manifestly transmitted through nature, sex, pregnancy, and birth, from one generation to another. It is now common knowledge that long-term narcotic exposure causes permanent change in the human brain and that heavy alcohol, tobacco, and cocaine use by mothers leads to various forms of defects among newborns.

Modes of Learning: Association versus Identification

There are various ways in which one learns substance use. An important contrast that distinguishes one method from another is association versus identification.

As explained in the original learning theory, association emphasizes direct, face-to-face contact. Users develop interest, attempt first use, practice essential skills, internalize certain motives, and become adapted to use in close interactions with experienced users. Experienced users may include family members, relatives, classmates, co-workers, and neighborhood buddies. Close interactions may range from living under one roof, playing in the same park, doing weekend excursions together, and studying in the same school, to following a similar routine in the community. Learning may involve observation, imitation, apprenticeship, formal instruction, and informal advice. For instance, an experienced user may teach a novice hand by hand and word by word from initiation to habitual use through formal apprenticeship. In a club or collective gathering, the organizer may ask for attention from all participating members and offer a quasi-professional seminar on a substance regarding its general properties, preparation procedures, steps of use, typical effects, and possible social reactions. A father may informally pass on a subtle use skill to his son when he says to him: "I do not think you should ever try it. But if you do, be sure not to mess it up with X or drink a cup of Y when you feel nauseous."

Identification, on the other hand, traces the effect of learning to the source of learning from which the learner may apparently remain distant but with which he or she may have become identified. In an age when telecommunications bring the world together, when mass media play a pervasive role in everyday life, and when information, fashion, and vogue spread instantly, distant, virtual, or identification learning seems to become more and more common, powerful, and effective than its close, direct, or association counterpart. First, substance users can easily develop interests, motives, and justifications to use from celebrities, the rich, the powerful, or the famous, featured regularly in mass media. They ask: if some of our national leaders experimented with drugs when they were young, why not me during my adolescence or early adulthood? Second, users can handily obtain information about cultivation, preparation, use, and effect management from various sources, including academic materials, prevention brochures, websites, and Internet chatrooms. One does not have to intern in a plantation or laboratory if he or she wants to grow marijuana or make amphetamines. He or she just needs to buy a manual or download some information from the World Wide Web, and follow the directions provided in those materials. Third, a drug subculture that has miraculously developed and enduringly sustained amid the constant flow of information, commercialism, and social rebellion provides support for whoever can identify with it by whatever means. For example, one can naturally pitch into the up-and-down use cycle of a substance when he or she just keeps watching news, seeing movies, reading underground circulars or regular publications, and visiting some feature websites.

Content of Learning: Motive versus Technique

What specifics do users need to learn pertaining to substance use? From users to user groups, from substances to substance properties, from use effects to symptom management, and from social controls of substance use to subcultural strategies by users, there are obviously numerous sketches or details to know for any common users. On substances and substance properties, for example, users may need to not only gain general information about different types of substances and subtypes of a substance, but also acquire specific knowledge about a type or subtype of a substance regarding its unique supply, purity, market form, preparation, use procedure, and user effects.

On a general level, learning for substance users can break down into two parts: motives and techniques. Motives include moral explanations, justifications, and rationalizations developed among existing users and in the current substance subculture in response to self- and social questioning, condemnations, and attacks. Before use, prospective users learn to clear up concerns, overcome fears, develop interests, and build up motivations for actual onset to substance use. They typically reason: nothing bad will happen; I will not be caught; and I will not become hooked to the substance. During use, users learn to accept changed consciousness or feelings, justify enhanced or reduced mental ability and social functionality, and rationalize the nuances, disruption, or damages they occasionally cause in the family, workplace, and neighborhood. They usually argue: use is fun; it is okay to skip work once in a while; and it is not so terrible as I used to think to be questioned by the police. After a certain period of use, users learn to explain habitual use, defend dependency or association with experienced users, and glorify use, disruptive behavior, and nonproductive lifestyle with systematic inputs from the substance subculture. They may assert: use is beneficial; users are not junkies but people of higher conscience, honesty, and morality; it is better to be an outsider from the mainstream society because the so-called mainstream society becomes increasingly unfair, unjust, and meaningless.

Techniques, in contrast, involve the technological aspects of substance use. Although not every user has to become an expert on every link, there are skills and techniques to be learned and improved in the whole sequence of substance use. First regards supply. How does one obtain his or her substance in good quality, at a reasonable price, and under minimal risk? An accurate judgment on quality requires observational subtlety, tasting sharpness, and familiarity with a substance and its various types and market forms. A bargain in price results from calculative negotiation. Risks may come from law enforcement officials as well as drug dealers. They can be minimized if users know whom they deal with, where, when, and how to best deal with them. Second regards preparation. Users may need to cut the raw materials into different parts, divide the substance into proper dosages, and put it into ready-to-use forms. They may need to change the physical form of the substance from solid to liquid to a gaseous state. They may need to dilute the dosage with certain liquids, mix the substance with some other materials, and place the final preparation in a syringe or other paraphernalia. They may even learn to engage in some chemical procedures to change the molecular composition of a substance. For example, freebasing cocaine users treat street cocaine with a liquid base, such as buffered ammonia, to change it from the salt form to a base form. They then dissolve the base cocaine in a solvent, such as ether, to obtain purified crystals, which they crush to use in a special heated glass pipe (Inciardi 1992). Some marijuana smokers use their preferred substance in the form of blunts. In preparing blunts, they first take a cigar, slit it open, and empty out all the tobacco. They then put herbs in it, roll it up, lick it, seal it, and make it ready for use.

Third concerns use. There are different ways to take a substance: inhaling, swallowing, drinking, smoking, or injecting. Each method of administration has its unique features. For example, injection may take a substance into the body subcutaneously, intramuscularly, or intravenously (Doweiko 1996). In injection, users may empty a whole syringe of substance once in a second, intermittently during a certain period, or gradually over a considerable time. Most important, users learn to perceive, sense, and enjoy the effects of the substance while avoiding being irritated, choking, fainting, or becoming intoxicated due to improper intake. Fourth relates to effect management. While some instant effects during use may appear to be euphonious and pleasurable, users sooner or later have to face withdrawal symptoms, chemical dependency, tolerance reactions, feelings of craving, side effects, and other problematic experiences from substance use. To sustain the habit, they need to learn both general strategies and specific tactics in response to all possible situations and scenarios. Finally, users may have a natural interest in gathering information about treatment facilities and user support groups. This happens when they are occasionally brought to a facility for emergency treatment or they voluntarily seek help for some of their urgently felt problems.

With proper motives and techniques learned in sufficient proficiency, users may be able to speak a whole language of substance use. Specifically, they know and understand a special argot or lingo pertaining to certain substances in particular and all substance use in general. For example, marijuana users may talk about pot, weed, herb, joints, blunts, chronic, green, cess, skunk, red hair, hydro, chocolate Thai, homegrown, stress weed, and other jargon or slang specific to the substance. Cocaine users may call their preferred substance shit, coke, bernice, Big C, corrine, lady snow, toot, nose candy, or Super Fly, while people in the crack circle may use castles, base houses, brothels, residence houses, resorts, or graveyards to refer to places where crack is prepared, sold, and used (Inciardi 1992). By using special terms and idioms, substance users not only obtain a verbal shorthand to summarize complex ideas and meanings among themselves, but also secure a means of safeguard to promote group cohesiveness and provide boundary maintenance in exclusion of outsiders (Sebald 1968).

Stages of Learning: Interest versus Experience

Like learning other behaviors, learning substance use involves a process of sequential development. Prospective users first develop interest in a substance and become willing to try it. They then make their debut to use and experiment with the substance as a novice. At the third stage, they internalize user morality, broaden and sharpen use in terms of types, forms, methods, and skills, and join the rank of regular or habitual users. Next, they start to face and learn to deal with various problems associated with use. The last stage comes when users have traversed the whole spectrum of substance use. Drawing upon their learned experience, they may become entrepreneurs to operate a drug-dealing network or run substance-related services. They may rise to the role of educators to take novice users under their apprenticeship or teach prospective users to stay away from drugs. They may even serve as role models to highlight the glamor and benefit of substance use among potential and existing users or encourage addicts to recover from drug dependency.

Obviously, the sequential development of learning corresponds to, as well as interacts with, the natural progression of substance use, from initiation, to experimentation, to habituation, to dependency, and to abstinence, as dictated by the effect of the substance, the adaptation of the user, and the reaction from the user's social environment. Initiation is usually prompted by such factors as an exposure to substance use scenes, a dissatisfaction with the existing state of affairs, and an association with substance users. Once users come to perceive substance use as a way out of their personal malaise and view themselves as capable of controlling their substance use, they start to experiment with a full variety of use in terms of the substance consumed and the method adopted. Experimentation paves the way to habituation. During habituation, users fine-tune specific techniques, rationalize use and related behaviors, and develop their own use rituals, styles, and routines. After some experiences with dependency and abstinence, users may not only know how to prepare for or react to various possible problematic situations resulting from use, but also understand that there are both positive and negative aspects to substance use. With a balanced view, they may sooner or later realize that they have to make a choice between fascination and practical utility, between benefit and harm, and between use and nonuse.

An important contrast that persists through the learning process is interest versus experience. On the one hand, interest is driven by motives whereas experience builds mainly upon techniques. On the other hand, interest leads to the acquisition of experience, and experience in turn may fuel or provide guidance for one's interest to learn. In sequential development, users seem to first cultivate their motives for a substance and then learn various skills to use it. Once they use it, they tend to develop all necessary justifications and rationalizations pertaining to its use. With clear and specific justifications, they may move further to learn more sophisticated procedures, practice more refined techniques, and hence become more experienced users. Of course, experience may also serve as one's reason for quitting: "I have had it all. I have had it enough. It is time to stop it and start a new life."

Contingencies of Learning: Reinforcement versus Punishment

In the original learning theory, contingencies of learning fall simply into rewards and penalties. The presence of rewards or the absence of penalties reinforces learning, whereas the absence of rewards or the presence of penalties discourages learners from continuing their pursuits.

As far as substance use is concerned, rewards may range from physical pleasure, heightened euphoria, illusion from reality, acceptance into a group, speaking a lingo, a sense of belonging, and a perceived new identity, to a valid excuse from active social responsibilities. Penalties, in contrast, may include intoxication, withdrawal symptoms, craving, tolerance reactions, dependency, family pressures, financial strains, police arrests, layoffs, and a loss of social status. While it is generally true that rewards tend to push users further into use and penalties are likely to pull users away from their habit, it is possible that they each work in the opposite way, pending when, where, and how they act upon what kind of users with what kind of self-perception. For instance, a hangover, when it is experienced by a first-time user, may serve as a reason for further use. However, when it is projected by a second-time user, a hangover may loom as a penalty against any idea of use. Similarly, the image of chemical dependency may scare people from ever experimenting with drugs, whereas the situation of actual addiction usually exists as an entrapment to keep users in continual use and dependency.

In addition to the consequential rewards or penalties emerging naturally from the process of use, two socially instituted contingencies, prevention and intervention, are often introduced to change the balance between learning and unlearning. Prevention targets prospective users. It aims to arm people with information and images about substance use and its various penalizing consequences so that they voluntarily avoid use and stay abstinent from drugs. Intervention, on the other hand, focuses on existing users. It intends to provide them with tangible benefits and support so that they choose to give up use and return to the normal way of life. From a dialectical point of view, however, perceived penalties may also prompt people to adventure into the risk of use while experienced rewards do not always overcome users' entrenched dependence upon a substance. Learning, unlearning, and their respective positive or negative reinforcement are all contingent upon various contingencies, which are themselves contingent upon a web of other social and personal conditions.

The Context of Learning: Subculture versus Social Atmosphere

Learning substance use takes place in informal associations and formal groups, specific situations and general environments, as well as particular moods and universal sentiments. Informal associations range from parties, picnics, evening bars, night clubs, camps, and homeless clusters, to street gangs, while formal groups include families, kinships, schools, employment organizations, and other well-established institutions. Specific situations may prompt or prohibit substance use, whereas general environments may discourage or encourage users to develop their drug habits. For instance, within the context of a family, parents may have successfully cultivated in the minds of their children a strong antiuse attitude, but one child's failure in school and exposure to marijuana use in the neighborhood may still grow into a learning situation in favor of use. Sanctions imposed by parents and attention given by other family members may serve to reinforce the child to make steady progress in his or her acquisition of use motives and skills. Similarly, particular moods refer to various pro- or antiuse feelings held by different groups in specific situations, while universal sentiments reflect the prevailing reaction toward substance use by a society across its whole system and over time. In the United States, for example, although a war on drugs has long and consistently been fought, a multitude of interest groups still exist to promote use, advocate for legalization, and protect their unique use moods and situations in the service of their specific constituencies.

Among all the opposing contexts of learning, the contrast between subculture and social atmosphere is most representative and illustrative. Substance use subculture is a permeative but centripetal social phenomenon. On the one hand, it resides in family, school, and community; it accompanies youth, adults, and the elderly or artists, health professionals, and technocrats; and it penetrates the media, language, and daily communications. On the other hand, it gathers and spreads detailed information on substances; it rigorously and persistently promotes substance use; and it meticulously serves users in their specific needs. Within the substance use subculture, users can learn through association or identification; they can learn motives or techniques; and they can learn step by step, progressing from interested novices to experienced masters. For instance, one first experiments with marijuana with his or her schoolmates. But it is through media, literature, growers' networks, and users' clubs embodying the marijuana use subculture that he or she learns all specific justifications, techniques, and skills pertaining to cultivation, shipment, storage, preparation, use, and effect management.

While substance use subculture as reflected in specific settings provides users with concrete learning tasks and devices, social atmosphere determines the extent substance use subculture expands to and impacts upon the whole cultural system. In the time when a strong antiuse sentiment persists through the general population, substance use subculture may only survive as an underground counterculture. In the time when use mixes with nonuse in a seemingly unclear contrast between harms and benefits, substance use subculture may become immersed in the general culture as an inseparable element. Ironically in contemporary society, as more and more people experience ambivalence toward knowledge and common sense, health and pleasure, renovation and rebellion, diversity and simplicity, and various other contradictions in life, substance use and its subculture seem to be gaining lifts from both sides of the contrast. For instance, the war on drugs may have helped to glorify the image of users as well as to diversify the vocabulary for use justification. After years of war on drugs, now in the general social atmosphere, not only do users appear to be "braver, smarter, tougher, more adventurous, or more rebellious," but also use seems to be "more understandable, excusable, tolerable, and acceptable."

Theoretical Applications

Applying the social learning perspective, a variety of theoretical questions can be raised regarding users as learners, substances as subjects of learning, and uses as learned behaviors.

Beginning with users, are they experiential or intellectual learners? Experiential learners develop a habit of use through association with parents, relatives, classmates, workmates, and peers, while intellectual learners learn how to use a substance from the mass media, fads and vogues, and literary sources by way of identification. Are they morally or technically oriented learners? Morally oriented learners focus on motives, rationalizations, and justifications, whereas technically oriented learners emphasize techniques, skills, and workmanship pertaining to substance use. Are they fast, steady, and experienced or slow, unstable, and delinquent learners? A fast, steady, and experienced learner may have mastered all essential skills after a few experimentations, while a slow, unstable, and delinquent learner may have never internalized use morality and technicality over a long period of irregular exposure. Also, are some learners more susceptible to reinforcement than others? Are some learners more capable of unlearning use than others? For instance, prevention, legal intervention, and medical treatment may lead some users to abstinence, cessation, and recovery while prompting or plunging other users into initiation, experimentation, relapse, and addiction.

As far as substances are concerned, are they classified or unclassified? Classified substances may necessitate a considerable technicality in their acquisition and consumption. Are they licit or illicit substances? Illicit substances may involve a complex justification system for their use. Are they popular or relatively unknown substances? A popular substance may attract a large number of novices to experiment with it. Learning its use may therefore become a social vogue. Are they club drugs, partner drugs, or loners' drugs? Some drugs appear and become available in clubs and social gatherings. People learn how to use them and continue to use them in specific group activities in particular group settings. Are they gateway substances or hard drugs? Gateway substances usually lay a foundation, in both use motives and techniques, for onset to hard drugs. In addition, the level of tolerance, the power of dependency, the severity of withdrawal, and other substance-specific characteristics may influence who learns, what is learned, as well as where, when, and how learning occurs and progresses.

The environment of learning consists of various forces and conditions on three levels: community, culture, and historical era. At the level of community, how readily available are substances, substance use devices, and substance venues? To what extent are users connected to one another? To what degree are they motivated to sanctify and perpetuate their substance use lifestyle through recruitment and apprenticeship? At the level of culture, how is substance use perceived by the general public? How are substance users portrayed in the mass media? What legal regulations and sanctions are instituted on substance use? Are there moral and legal contrasts between the mainstream that restricts substance use and a subculture that promotes substance use? Finally, a historical era may be marked by tolerance or intolerance for substance use, control or legalization of certain substances, and a high or low level of substance use, misuse, and dependency. All these can obviously affect learning, learners, and learned behaviors in substance use and abuse.

Empirical Tests

The social learning perspective is amenable to empirical tests using different research methods. Empirical studies of learning with respect to its learners, content, conditions, contingencies, contexts, and outcomes provide opportunities to sharpen and improve various research tools as well.

Case studies focus on individual learners or substances. Each individual user is unique because he or she may develop his or her own learning story in terms of a single learning variable. For instance, one user demonstrates an extraordinary influence of identification in learning while another exhibits a curvilinear learning path in response to rewards and penalties from the environment. A multitude of case studies may converge to show a general pattern for users, substances, or a learning variable. For instance, young users learn more and faster by way of identification in the era of mass media and cyberspace communications. Association takes effect mostly with a lead figure. Or substance X is favored by and learning of its usage spreads mainly among transsexuals, the homeless, clubgoers, or dandies.

Survey research asks users questions about their learning experience. Information can be gathered representatively or unrepresentatively about a population, a substance, or any aspect of learning. Regarding a population, how is use transmitted from one section, ethnic group, age cohort, or generation to another? How are users distributed in terms of learning abilities or outcomes? Is there a substance use subculture? How is the substance subculture related to the learning of substance use? Regarding a substance, is it difficult to gain access to its user group? Is it easy to learn its use? Are there sophisticated procedures to follow in the acquisition of its complex use techniques or its specific use justifications? What makes the substance typically a substance of learning through stages, by way of association, or without relevance to reinforcement? In terms of learning itself, questions may be included to explore stages of learning, contents of learning, as well as relative influences of association, identification, or reinforcement and their respective agents. For instance, why is association more powerful than identification? Why are peers more influential than parents for certain substances or among some users?

Experimental studies are useful and effective in examining how learning is impacted by reinforcement conditions in different types, schedules, and intensities. In controlled experiments, subjects may be given varying dosages of a substance on a varying schedule with or without relieving medications for withdrawal symptoms to see how they learn and adapt to the casual or habitual use of the substance. By quasi-experimental design, subjects may be divided into groups with or without exposure to some specific reinforcers, such as prevention materials, drug-using peers, or prodrug propaganda, to determine whether learning is facilitated or hindered by those reinforcement conditions. Quasi-experimental research may also be used to explore the effects of various other factors on the process of learning. For instance, parents, role models, peers, the media, the subculture, and other association or identification variables can each be scrutinized in comparative conditions of absence versus presence to ascertain their respective weight in the learning of substance use.

POLICY IMPLICATIONS

On the policy front, the social learning perspective provides ideas and insights that might inform a more intellectual, rational, scientific, and learned approach, strategy, practice, or social action plan for substance use and abuse.

Public Health

Viewing users as learners, public health professionals need to tackle two important tasks. On the one hand, they need to engage in serious scientific research and clinical trials to obtain accurate and systematic information and knowledge about various substances being used and abused by certain groups or across the general population. Medical researchers study pharmaceutical properties of each substance, its chemical structure, physiological functions, and neurobiological effects. Clinical physicians study users of a substance. They observe symptoms, make diagnoses, and develop treatment plans. Nursing staff enforce treatments, record reactions, and care for patients in the process of recovery. Together, scientists and practitioners in health and medicine are responsible for the validity and reliability of all essential information and knowledge available for each substance, its chemical features, use effects, use prevalence, user characteristics, and user treatment regimens.

On the other hand, public health officials and professionals need to ensure that existing information and knowledge about substance and substance use are disseminated objectively and in a timely manner to both specific targets and the general public. Just as funding is essential to scientific research in obtaining knowledge, financial support is indispensable to prevention and education as a means to spread knowledge. In prevention and education, it is important that different channels and forums, from mass media to public schools, from family to community, and from public venues to workplaces, are utilized to reach different segments of the population, from the rich to the poor, from the literate to the illiterate, from the mainstream to the underground, and from the conventional to the deviant. It is even more important that information is presented to the audience objectively, straightforwardly, and honestly. There is no intent to cause scare, panic, and shame among recipients on the part of information providers.

With ready access to reliable knowledge, people can make a learned choice about their substance use. Health professionals can therefore spare some of their traditional efforts in conventional prevention and treatment.

Social Control

Knowing that people learn substance use and that their learning can be modified through rewards and penalties, social control agents need to make some adjustments on their often taken-for-granted reactions to substance, substance use, and substance users.

First, learning on each substance progresses with science and technology. Classification and subsequent control of a substance should not only be based on knowledge but also remain responsive to most updated learning from scientific research. A new substance, when it first appears on the market, should not automatically be placed under control simply because it belongs to a family of classified substances by chemical structure or some pharmaceutical properties. Instead, decisions on its classification and control should be based on a series of scientific and clinical studies on all aspects of the substance and its usage. A substance that is currently under control, if it is found to be beneficial for medical use or not as addictive or threatening as it was previously thought by mounting recent research, should be taken out of the classification system for scientific experimentation, clinical trials, and further regulated or unregulated use by needed or interested users. Similarly, some widely used substances, if they are proved by sufficient empirical evidence to be serious health and safety hazards, may be classified for regulation and control.

Second, rules, laws, and sanctions regarding substance and substance use are made systematically, written in clear language, and publicized through known media. With regulations well publicized, people know what they can do and what they cannot do, and become prepared for any legal and social consequences that may result from their chosen substance use. Written in clear language, regulations can not only be easily understood by people who are concerned with substance use, but also be less vulnerable to misinterpretations by attorneys and judges in the court procedure. Finally, a systematic regulatory system gives people opportunities to weigh different options and make the most appropriate choices in their substance use. For instance, some may retreat to using only the least regulated substance while a few may simplify their use to the most controlled drug.

Third, social control agents act responsibly, consistently, professionally, and effectively in accordance with the law. The key is consistency. Consistency teaches people that there is no chance to avoid penalties or to not face consequences. Inconsistency, on the other hand, may implicitly encourage people to test the water. For instance, youths would attempt to buy cigarettes or frequent bars if they knew they would not always be asked for identification. Merchants would not be willing to lose sales or bartenders be willing to lose tips if they learned they did not have to worry about police detection and customer report all the time. More subtly, random lax or drastic measures taken by the authority toward certain substances, using places, or using activities may unnecessarily mislead users to escalation and other problem behaviors. For example, marijuana use becoming a vogue, crack houses moving underground, and intravenous heroin injection being specialized through shooting galleries may to some degree reflect inconsistency, irrationality, intolerance, lapse, or connivance inherent in social control reactions to substance use and abuse.

Life and Community

Substance use takes place in the community. Substance users learn and unlearn use amid routine activities in daily life. With a social learning perspective, efforts can be made pointedly to change substance use through sources, contingencies, and a milieu of learning.

Family, school, gang, peer group, and other community-based networks provide major sources of learning in substance use. While living with a smoker under the same roof, studying with a marijuana user in the same classroom, or playing with a designer drug experimenter in the same community park prompts learning through association, seeing a beauty smoking or a celebrity drinking on neighborhood billboards, watching drug dealers cruising in luxury cars, or sensing some substance-related fads going on in local clubs may activate learning through identification. To prevent or reduce substance use, agents or factors of learning in both association and identification dimensions need to be addressed throughout life and the community.

Parental disciplining, academic evaluation, peer recognition, and membership in certain local groups may serve as contingencies of learning for substance use. Restrictive parenting may create children's needs for attention and freedom through substance use while permissiveness by parents may leave children with both money and leeway in experimenting with drugs. Failure in school may lead to deviations in the form of substance use but celebrations over positive academic performance may also supply reasons for drinking, smoking, and even trying hard drugs. Some experimenting drug users may be reinforced to progress into habitual or problematic use when they are made to believe, by a temporary performance in school, that they can hide and manage their use without obvious detrimental consequences. Peer recognition and membership in certain groups work similarly in terms of use initiation, escalation, and habituation. It is therefore important to cover all contingencies inherent in various aspects of life and the community regarding substance use prevention and intervention.

Finally, the general environment, as demonstrated by residents' attitudes, the neighborhood's physical outlook, and various territorial groups' activities, may deter or prompt substance use in the community. In a community where the majority of residents hold a liberal attitude toward a substance, such as marijuana, the substance may be publicly grown in the backyard, processed in the basement, and used in gatherings for all locals. In a neighborhood where there is a heavy presence of bars, liquor stores, night clubs, graffiti, and billboard advertisements for alcohol, tobacco, and other substances, people may feel natural or even pressured to engage in use. In an area where school is dysfunctional, unemployment is high, gangs reign by terror, and the police patrol in high alert, drug dealing and substance use may coexist as one of the social diseases therein. To prevent and reduce substance use, it is often necessary to reform, reinvent, and rejuvenate a whole community in all its aspects, from educational access, employment opportunities, public amenities, and recreational activities, to neighborhood sanitation, order, health, and appearance.

Work and Organization

Given the importance of work and the prevalence of organizational employment in contemporary time, work and organization can be a powerful reinforcement for learning or unlearning substance use through both association and identification.

First, learning or unlearning through association can go hand in hand with that through identification. The former occurs by itself when employees learn from each other in employee lounges, cafeterias, or work positions within the organization and their children learn from one another in the same school, club, or community park serving the organization. It mixes with the latter, learning through identification with people in higher position or social status, when one learns to use a substance because his or her boss uses the substance and when one's child learns to use a substance because he looks up to the boss's child as a model in use of the substance. Beyond a particular employment organization, identification may even play a primary role in motivating people to learn substance use across an occupation or profession. For instance, one picks up the habit of using one substance because one of his or her most respected fellow professionals is known to use the substance.

Second, experiences at work, both positive and negative, may serve as causes for substance use. While problematic relations, lagging performance, warnings, disciplinary actions, demotion, suspension, and loss of employment may drag people into use and abuse, celebrations over salary increase, promotion, and other job awards may give people reasons for a drinking spree or some special treatments with some special substances, such as a name-brand liquor, imported tobacco products, or a designer drug. In terms of reinforcement, substance use may affect job performance, job performance produces differential awards or penalties, and awards or penalties at work may directly or indirectly act on use, sending it into escalation, modification, or termination. On the other hand, drug violations may lead to criminal justice actions, criminal justice actions may result in demotion, suspension, or expulsion from work, and loss of essential interest in employment may further complicate use, making it a temporary escape or even a final retreat from productive social life.

Third, work and organizations may provide access to, incentives for, and a learning environment of substance use. Alcohol and tobacco are necessary elements in a variety of business dealings, such as receptions, conference banquets, contract-signing ceremonies, grand openings, and employee retreats. Some specialty employees, including negotiators, product sales representatives, and those in public relations, may have to intentionally train themselves to improve their ability to consume alcohol and/or tobacco. In China, for example, many successful salesmen from manufacturing companies are capable drinkers at the dinner table where business deals are negotiated and sealed. More common and seemingly casual than alcohol and tobacco, coffee and tea are provided in many workplaces around the world. Employees are implicitly or explicitly lured or educated to use them amid the excitement, stress, or boredom of their work routine. In special occupations and professions that are involved in growing, manufacturing, processing, shipping, dispensing, or controlling certain substances, knowledge learned and access gained through job or in the workplace about those substances may prompt some employees or professionals into use and abuse. For instance, some medical professionals use drugs not only because they have ready access to drugs, but also because they feel they know more than other people about drugs and therefore have better control over drug use (Coombs 1997).

Knowing all these connections to substance use and its learning, appropriate policies can be made and modified in work and organizational settings to assist drug-using employees in their struggle toward recovery and to motivate employers in their efforts in prevention and intervention.

In sum, the social learning perspective brings a unique view and approach to substance, substance use, and substance users. Knowledge on substance changes with science and technology. It is unevenly and unequally distributed over the population and through generations. A substance is used in a society often because it is known to that society. It is abused in a society sometimes because it is not so well understood by and hence remains a myth to that society. On the individual level, some people use and misuse a substance out of misinformation, misunderstanding, and ignorance while others do so due to a seemingly well-informed, well-educated, and well-polished professional background.

Substance use is a learned behavior. A society passes its knowledge as well as its habit of use, misuse, or abuse of a substance from time to time. Individuals learn about a substance and its use, misuse, or abuse from parents, relatives, neighbors, classmates, co-workers, or peers through association. They also learn from the literature, the mass media, myth, or hearsay by way of identification. Learning can be casual, gradual, and in the context of other activities or formal, focused, and in exclusion of all life commitments. Things learned usually include interests, motives, justifications, skills, techniques, and precautions regarding a substance, its use, and consequences from its use. While there might be a system of information about all aspects of use pertaining to a substance, most people learn it step by step, piece by piece. The acquisition, mastery, and utilization of knowledge and experience about a substance and its use are always differentially graded across any given user population.

Substance users are learners. Although they begin with different abilities and capacities, they are essentially influenced or dictated by whom they are associated with, whom they become identified with, what moral messages they are exposed to, what technical complexities they are taught with, what rewards they are given, what penalties they are threatened with or face, and what subculture they are thrown into in the process of learning and sustaining substance use. With proper changes in internal motivation and external pressure, users may learn to exit from or unlearn substance use by modes, through stages, under contingencies, and in contexts similar to those of learning.

The unique view taken by the social learning perspective not only informs academic, policymaking, social control, and social service communities of new ideas and new ways of thinking, but also warns them of a practical need to take a learning and learned approach toward their respective work on substance, substance use, and substance users.

—9—

The Social Reaction Perspective

Substance use is a social phenomenon. Analogous to a theater play where actors and actresses perform acts in response to the reactions from the audience, substance users choose or avoid, escalate or lessen, modify or routinize, and abandon or maintain substance use on the basis of the various inputs they receive from their living environments.

The social reaction perspective capitalizes on the interactive nature of the three-way relations among substance users (actor), substance use (act), and societal responses (audience). It attempts to describe and explicate how one shapes and is shaped by another in a cyclical sequence involving all three variables. Beginning with substance use, for example, the social reaction perspective explores and explains why it is initiated, pursued, and cherished or avoided, resisted, and hated by actual and prospective users, why it is prompted, sanctified, and perpetuated or prohibited, stigmatized, and eliminated by society, and most essentially, how societal reactions implicitly and explicitly influence the way users see and behave themselves, the way they view and continue their substance use, and the way they perceive and approach life, work, society, and the whole world.

SOURCES OF INSPIRATION

The social reaction perspective traces its theoretical roots to some of the early ideas in social psychology. Charles Horton Cooley (1902) coined the concept of looking-glass self to explain his observation that an individual's self-evaluation and self-identity are basically a reflection of one's perception of other people's reactions to his or her conduct. W. I. Thomas (1931) put forth the famous proposition that when people define a situation as real, it becomes real in its consequence, in his thought-provoking theory on the definition of the situation. Later, Robert Merton (1968) developed the idea of self-fulfilling prophecy. According to him, when members of a social group define a person or event in certain ways, they may so shape future activities and circumstances to give way to their anticipated and projected behaviors.

The publication of *Crime and the Community* by Frank Tannenbaum in 1938 represents the formal establishment of a social reaction perspective in the field of deviance and criminology. By studying the societal treatment of offenders, Tannenbaum (1938) discovered a gradual shift, or a process of tagging, "from the definition of the specific acts as evil to a definition of the individual as evil" (17). He argued that as "the person becomes the thing he is described as being" (20), the societal treatment makes hardened criminals out of accidental or occasional ones. The greater evil, thus, lies in the societal treatment, not the original act.

The landmark contribution to the modern labeling approach, however, was made by Edwin Lemert (1951). Lemert was primarily concerned with labeling as a critical determinant of the subsequent deviant or conforming career of an individual. Building on Tannenbaum's (1938) implicit progression from the first act to the final behavior, he made an explicit distinction between primary and secondary deviations. Primary deviation occurs when an individual commits one or several deviant acts, but does not internalize the deviant self-concept and continues to occupy the role of conformist. Secondary deviation, in contrast, occurs when an individual assumes the deviant role imputed to him or her through societal reactions and behaves in accordance with his or her so-altered self-concept. For instance, a juvenile is formally labeled by the court as a delinquent. When he comes home from a juvenile incarceration facility, he feels that his parents, relatives, neighbors, schoolmates, and everybody else in the community look at him differently as if he were a troublemaking demon. He then starts to think of himself as a delinquent and wonder what a delinquent would do under various circumstances. The subsequent law-violating behaviors he commits become secondary deviations as he actively hangs out with other delinquent youth and seeks to meet the expectations required by his newly acquired deviant identity.

Following Lemert's work, the labeling or social reaction perspective is applied to a wide range of issues in crime, deviance, and criminal justice. Howard Becker (1963) studied marijuana users and introduced the notion of a developmental process that moves from attainment of a deviant identity to devoted participation in a deviant career. Irving Piliavin and Scott Briar (1964) examined police/juvenile encounters and found that many dispositions made by police officers in cases of suspected juvenile offenders are made "often on the basis of the public face he has presented to officials rather than the kind of offense he has committed" (214). Aaron

Cicourel (1968) reviewed files kept by schools, police departments, and courts about individual youth and discovered that ad hoc interpretations of character, family life, and future possibilities by those authority agencies not only negatively label some juveniles, but also literally predispose them to future litigation. Edwin Schur (1973) documented the overuse of stigmatizing labels in juvenile justice and insisted that so-called delinquents are neither internally nor externally different from nondelinquents except for the fact that they have been officially processed by the justice system. Hugh Barlow (1987) noticed the distinction between acts of mala in se (considered inherently evil) and mala prohibita (considered evil only because they are prohibited) and claimed that a wide variety of acts become treated as status offenses not because they are evil in and of themselves, but merely because they have been labeled as inappropriate behavior for juveniles. Recently, David Ward and Charles Tittle (1993) pointed out that "sanctioning and labeling of norm violators significantly affects the likelihood that an offender will develop a deviant identity and that such identities significantly affect the likelihood of recidivism" (60).

In substance abuse research, subtle changes in individual attitude, perspective, and behavior are first revealed among marijuana users by Howard Becker's pioneer study. According to Becker (1963), becoming a confirmed and consistent user of marijuana involves three related steps. Each step requires explanation. "We need, for example, one kind of explanation of how a person comes to be in a situation where marijuana is readily available . . . and another kind of explanation of why, given the fact of its availability, he is willing to experiment with it in the first place. And we need still another explanation of why, having experimented with it, he continues to use it" (23). However, a study commissioned by the National Institute on Drug Abuse asserted that the commitment of the marijuana user is highly variable, ranging from the minimal commitment of experimentation to the firm commitment of habituation. With regard to the change in self-identity, it pointed out that "current attitudes toward the drug laws and the lack of uniform enforcement tend to aid the adolescent in seeing themselves a 'victim' of an unjust system. Such a view could act as a neutralizing device against threats to the self-concept" (Williams 1976: 23).

On alcohol use, some studies confirm that people who are perceived as socially deviant, under the label of "problem drinker" or "alcoholic," tend to jeopardize their health by drinking excessively (Walton 1992). Some studies refute the hypothesis that being labeled an alcoholic results in poor drinking outcomes (Combs-Orme, Helzer, and Miller 1988). Florence Ridlon (1988) conducted research on how status insularity functions for female alcoholics. She argues that women are less likely than men to be labeled, that women will be more heavily stigmatized should they be labeled alcoholic, and that women are more likely than men to have lower self-esteem and suffer various forms of secondary deviation should they be more heavily stigmatized. Contrary to use, treatment for alcoholism emphasizes the critical importance of problem identification, often in the form of negative labels, toward assistance seeking and recovery. Alcoholics Anonymous (AA) begins with the member's self-admission as an alcoholic in need of help. Many clinical treatments by professionals follows a similar procedure in which the initial phase encompasses assessing problems, labeling the alcoholism, and devising a treatment contract (Usher 1991).

Regarding other substances and substance use in general, the process as well as the effect of labeling, delabeling, and relabeling through use, addiction, treatment, recovery, and abstinence are sporadically touched upon by a number of studies using specific data or targeting specific subjects and issues (Covington 1984; Ray and Downs 1986; Kaplan 1987; Kaplan and Fukurai 1992; Hassin 1994). Jay Williams (1976) noted that the use of LSD or heroin seems more heinous than the use of marijuana in the public and official view. Focusing on the effect of arrest and identification of an adolescent "addict" or "drug abuser" on his or her self-image and subsequent behavior, he finds that "official labelers may well provide an adolescent with a positive label in his reference peer group rather than with the intended negative label whose reference is the larger conventional society" (23). Jerry Meints (1979) conducted a large evaluation of a methadone program and established a model that explains rehabilitative success as a function of delabeling the heroin addict and relabeling him or her as a methadone patient. As Meints points out, the process of de- and relabeling operates to neutralize the stigma of prior drug-related arrests and facilitate social acceptance and subsequent social functioning. Interestingly, especially to people in education, media, and prevention, a recent study in New York City reveals that the diffusion of the idea "crack head" into drug subcultures and the stigmatized status attached to it appear to have protected some young adults from using cocaine (Furst, Johnson, Dunlap, and Curtis 1999).

THEORETICAL FRAMEWORK

Substance use is not just an individual behavior based upon individual free will. In the sense that an individual makes his or her choices in interaction with other social members and individual behaviors are shaped by larger social forces, substance use is a social act symbolizing general morale and sentiment in a society.

Definition

The social reaction perspective focuses on the interaction between individuals and society, between personal perception and public definition, and between individual choices and social actions. Inherent in the perspective are a sequence of process-embedded propositions. First, society imputes different values to different acts or deeds by individuals. Second, individuals tend to enhance their status by pursuing different things ranked for differential social significance. Third, a substance is used in the way that it is socially defined and perceived as a symbol of defiance, rebellion, or distinction or a means toward relief, pleasure, or transcendence. Fourth, people use a substance and become users when they are confirmed by social reactions with their initial expectations for the substance. Fifth, users stay with a substance and become addicts when they are recognized and labeled by various parties in their surroundings for their continual interest in the substance. Sixth, addicts wrestle with a substance and become troublemakers when they are identified and treated by various social agents for their chronic problems with the substance. Finally, troublemakers turn into social outcasts when they are marginalized and cast out by various institutional treatments or punishments for their helplessly enduring chemical dependency, deviance, or criminality.

Underlying the sequential development from users to addicts to troublemakers to social outcasts are four important conceptual milestones: status, labeling, perception, and subsequent behavior. Status is the prestige position one has in relation to others in one's social group. Labeling involves a process of communicating and recording status with indicative words. Perception refers to the effect that status is felt, understood, and accepted by one and one's group through the process of labeling. Subsequent behaviors are acts following the self-perceived internalization of specific status, labeling, and labels. Status progression in substance use and abuse clearly indicates that subsequent behaviors not only reinforce previous labeling and solidify previous status, but also lead to ever-compelling labeling, labels, and status.

Theoretical Image

Within the sphere of human interactions, nothing remains what it originally is and everything changes because of various forces around its origin, nature, social reaction, self-perception, and status.

Substances, at the outset, are determined by their chemical structure, pharmaceutical properties, and physiological functions. Poisons are poisons. They cannot be used as foods. Stimulants are stimulants. They cannot be called depressants. However, beyond the general categorization, substances are to a large extent defined by cultural, social, and historical forces. Although a substance does not change itself when it is negatively or positively identified, the labeling process works similarly as people use its social identification to feed back on their attitude and behavior toward the substance. Alcohol is alcohol. But it is different, in social perception

and therefore social reaction, from time to time, between when it is prohibited and when it is legalized, and from place to place, between where
it is promoted and where it is disallowed. Narcotics are narcotics. But they
are different, in social imagery and hence social consequence, from incident to incident, between when they are used by patients for pain relief
and when they are injected by intravenous users for pleasurable experience, and from occasion to occasion, between where they are administered
in medical clinics and where they are rotated through unsterilized needles
and syringes in shooting galleries. As an increasingly complicated system
is poised to divide substances into the controlled and the uncontrolled,
the licit and the illicit, or the mild and the severe, evils, sins, and crimi-
nalities are differentially created, assigned, and labeled in social imagery
and perception to various substances, even though some of them are com-
parably similar in their intoxication and addiction potency.

Substance users, supposedly, make choices upon their own "free will."
They know who they are and usually weigh the benefits versus harms
when they choose to use a substance. However, because they have a "free
will" to react and reflect upon what comes from their environment, substance users can be gradually and naturally drawn into some use state or
status they would never expect before. A middle-class professional who
initially drinks a cup of coffee on an occasional basis may not expect to
have incorporated caffeine intake into his or her daily routine after years
of work in a corporate environment where coffee is provided and drinking a cup of coffee becomes an opportunity for socializing, information
sharing, resting, or rejuvenating. As coffee drinking is so institutionalized,
habits, preferences, or rituals, such as "I drink only decaffeinated coffee,"
"John drinks coffee without sugar," or "Kelly prefers one brand to another" may become important labels, symbols, and guides for individuals to identify themselves and to connect with one another. Similarly, a
teenager who tries alcohol, tobacco, or marijuana out of curiosity may
never think ahead to what it might feel like to be a drinker, a smoker, or
a drug user. In fact, no matter how motivated he or she is, he or she does
not automatically acquire a status in the hierarchy of substance use. It is
usually through a long-evolving process that use is recognized for
labeling, a user is identified to bear labels, user identification is perceived
to modify self-evaluation, self-evaluation is internalized to act on use, and
use is intensified, stabilized, or perpetuated to qualify for a specific substance use status, either a social drinker or an alcoholic, a casual smoker
or a nicotine-dependent user, a recreational drug user or a drug addict.

While users obtain differential statuses in substance use through the
interactive process of individual motivation and choice versus social definition and reaction, a group, culture, or society as well as a period, generation, or era may analogously receive different reputations regarding the
level, intensity, and scope of substance use around the world or through-

out history. A group may promote some types of substances, specialize in some forms of use, or engage in some social advocacy for users with certain characteristics. When the group becomes widely known for its ideology and practice, it may be identified and labeled accordingly. The label may then stick to the group as group members and people who deal with the group become accustomed to using the label to guide their behavior toward the group. For instance, the United States is known for being the largest drug market in the world. The reputation is first created by the high level of drug demand, supply, transaction, and use in the country. But once it is established, dealers and users around the world may refer to it as a guide in their search for profit and subcultural support. U.S. law enforcement agents may follow it in their reflection and action upon drug dealing and use within their jurisdiction. So may mass media and the general public in the country. Similarly, if the current time is taken for granted by the populace or some underground and subcultural groups as a time of alcohol legalization, tobacco restriction, or marijuana liberalization, it may become natural for people to wonder: would it look premature if I cannot handle a can of beer? Would it smell bad when I breathe out tobacco-saturated air? Or would it look stubborn and unwise when I say harsh words about marijuana?

Theoretical Components

The social reaction perspective studies how social factors shape and reshape attitudes and behaviors by individuals. In substance use and abuse, as it is in deviance and crime, the social-individual interaction is epitomized in the process of labeling, delabeling, and relabeling.

Labeling

The attribution of an identifying label to an act or actor represents both the beginning and the end of the social-individual interactional process. As the beginning, it places a labeled individual into a specific mental and behavioral framework in which he perceives himself, and he fashions his social participation in accordance with the social expectation transmitted by the label. As the end, it concludes a social reaction process in which an individual is judged by his initial actions and deeds.

In substance use and abuse, there first is a hierarchy or a sequence of labels. People who hold an accommodating attitude toward drug use and users may be called drug sympathizers. People who make their initial onset to a substance may be called substance novices. Substance novices who experiment with different forms, dosages, and uses of a substance may be called experimenters. Experimenters who adopt a pattern of occasional recreational use may be called casual users. Experimenters and casual users who incorporate use into their regular routine may be called habitual users. Habitual users who depend upon the continual intake of a substance in their bodily functions may be called addicts. Addicts who create nuisances in their community may be called troublemakers. Troublemakers who cross the law may be identified as criminals. Addicts who assume a nonproductive lifestyle and put themselves under various heath risks may be called junkies. Obviously, a lower level of labeling in response to a lower degree of acts sets the stage for a higher intensity of use behavior, which in turn leads to qualification for a higher level of labels. In other words, the positive identification of a use status not only reinforces the existing use situation, but also tends to escalate it into a more severe stage. The dual effect of reinforcement and escalation applies similarly to users: as they take on what they are labeled, they move toward a higher user status.

Second, labeling can be made in effect not only by other people in society but also by substance users themselves. Under classic labeling theory, labels are first applied to the subjects who have been identified as offenders or law violators by society. They then internalize the identity as labeled and act accordingly thereafter. In substance use, however, not every use is formally identified and publicly labeled as a deviant, illegal, or criminal act. Nor is every user so identified as an immoral, law-violating, or offending actor. As a matter of fact, only a few controlled substances may trigger a formal process of arrest, prosecution, and punishment by the criminal justice system for those who use, possess, or deal them. The majority of substance users, including many illicit drug users, realize the extent, level, or severity of their use by themselves or through interactions with their family members, friends, and peers. Using labels they learn from the substance use subculture or public media, they may call themselves recreational drug users, alcoholics, or smokers, become identified with their so-labeled user status, and act accordingly in their subsequent use. For instance, one may use certain terms to proudly call him or herself an adventurous, distinguished, sophisticated, or high-class user when he or she is able to explore some innovative forms of use, attain a unique state of feelings, apply a combination of complex techniques, or gain access to a substance in its highest purity and potency.

Compared to labeling by others, self-labeling may provide a more powerful source of influence for identity acquisition, confirmation, and modification. Although labels used in self-labeling may emerge from formal or informal social interactions, acts or identities labeled usually fall under a domain that is missed by social order maintenance authorities owing to neglect, incompetency, or lack of regulation. For instance, some substances and their use are not currently regulated by law. Some substances and their use are so common that they are left to individual discretion. Some substances and their use are not considered harmful enough to warrant social intervention. As far as illicit drugs and their use are concerned, because the criminal justice system is incapable of identifying, labeling, and treating each of them in formal social sanctions, many users may label themselves into different use statuses and act accordingly on their own or with one another. The same is probably true for some highly skilled professional or hard-core criminals who win over the police and remain undeterred in their criminal undertakings.

Third, labeling may be carried on by a family from parents to children, creating a genealogical tradition of use for one, two, or several substances. The generational crossover of labeling is based upon commonsense perceptions, both by subjects themselves and by other ordinary people in their surroundings. For instance, a person from an alcoholic family may reason: "My father is an alcoholic. My grandfather was an alcoholic. Alcoholism has been with my family for a long time. I grew up with alcohol in my life. What am I supposed to do with alcohol when I feel I am an alcoholic by default?" Similarly, a person whose mother died of a crack overdose may take on an addict identity as he or she looks back into his or her family background: "I was born as a crack baby. My mother was a drug addict known to everyone in my life. I grew up with exposure to different types of drugs and different kinds of drug users. It is almost an automatic thing that I put on the shoes left by my mother."

While labeling crossover through generations may vary from substance to substance, family to family, and situation to situation, a generally applicable process can be visualized as follows: members in one generation are formally labeled as users or abusers; members in the following generation become gradually identified with the labels; internalized labels act on members of the current generation, channeling them into choices and behaviors designated by the labels; and acts taken by members of the current generation in line with the labels qualify them for formal labeling or a takeover of the labels earned by members of the previous generation. In contemporary society, scattered scientific evidence regarding the inheritable nature of alcoholism and other substance addictions can obviously reinforce generational crossover in labeling. So can the mass media as they rapidly spread scientific research, public opinions, and commonsense speculations across the population before serious rational and objective analysis, substantiation, and validation have ever taken place.

Fourth, labeling may be transmitted from one to another among peers, making some labels shared properties by a closely knit peer group. Like generational crossover, peer group spillover occurs when members of a group become identified with a label earned by the group or group leaders and act accordingly to qualify for the label by themselves. A typical scenario is: "All my friends smoke cigarettes. They are known smokers. I belong to my friends. I am part of them. I do not feel it right that I be an exception to the smoking reputation shared by my friends." In a more concrete situation, a person is brought to a club by his or her friends. Initially, he or she sits in the corner, listening to various voices and observing different activities. After several visits, he or she gradually gets adjusted to the club atmosphere. He or she realizes that his or her friends and other members of the club are users of a designer drug, as so understood and labeled by themselves as well as people in the community. Continuing to hang out with his or her friends and other members in the club, he or she gradually feels he or she is part of the club and shares the reputation it has in the eyes of both members and nonmembers. Upon this critical self-identification, he or she starts seriously learning and practicing all aspects of use of the designer drug. A period of time later, he or she becomes a full-fledged user, not only in name but also in reality.

Delabeling

Delabeling is apparently the opposite of labeling. Users give up use, clearing a user's label from themselves. Or in societal response terms, society formally takes off labels from users after a careful evaluation of their long-enough abstinence or recovery from use. For delabeling to take place, there are first a clear identification and a positive confirmation of the label or labels left by a formal labeling process. In twelve-step treatment, the first step one is required to take toward abstinence or delabeling is self-admission that he or she is an alcoholic or addict. Once the label is identified, delabeling can proceed with the subject dissociating from people and disengaging from activities so labeled. In the twelve-step process, although one associates with other alcoholics or addicts, he or she shares with them a strong intent to disengage from alcohol or drug use. As the previous discourse is reversed, the subject gradually walks into a new world. Delabeling completes when he or she assumes a new role and takes a new identity in the new world.

It is obvious that delabeling not only builds upon labeling, but also sets the stage for labeling. In the aforementioned process, a new label, such as "recovered addict," "nonuser," or "abstainer," is likely to be given the subject as he or she is fully delabeled from use or addiction. The dialectic relationship between labeling and delabeling is also epitomized in the sequential progression of use and user status where delabeling a lower level of use and user status leads further to the labeling of a higher level of use and user status. For instance, a progressive experimental user, as he or she is delabeled from experimental use, is labeled into habitual or problematic use.

Relabeling

Relabeling occurs in the sequential process of labeling for progressive users in the sense that labeling for a higher level of use involves delabeling from the lower status and hence relabeling with a new label suitable for the higher status. In a strict sense, however, relabeling means the simple restoration of a previously possessed or experienced fame or status. An abstaining user fails in fighting his or her withdrawal syndrome and swings back to use: he or she was a user and retakes his or her previous label as a user. A user succeeds in quitting his or her substance use and comes back to his or her long-forgotten abstinence: he or she used to be a nonuser and resumes his or her normal status as a nonuser.

In the whole spectrum of use explored and experienced by a user, he or she may constantly be delabeled from and relabeled into different user statuses as he or she faces changes in the type and potency of substances as well as ups and downs in the level, intensity, and consequence of use and abuse. For instance, along the common corridor from licit to illicit substances and from mild to hard drugs, one uses marijuana and comes back to marijuana as his or her drug of choice after a period of serious struggle with crack. With a particular substance, one uses methadone as a street drug and becomes a chronic methadone user later in clinical treatment after years of addiction to heroin. Among different types of substances, one is a speed user when he lives in the street. He stops using speed when he follows a helping couple to live for a period of time on their ranch where he occasionally uses marijuana amid light drinking and smoking. He uses speed again when he comes back to his homeless life in the city.

Underlying labeling, delabeling, and relabeling are three important variables. One is perception, a mental process that reflects upon labeling, translates it into human feelings, manifests changes in self-identity, and governs behavior subsequent to labeling and identity change. Another is primary substance use, an initial act that leads to social reaction or triggers formal labeling. Still another is secondary substance use, a progressive or regressive consequence that results from labeling and change in self-identity.

Perception

Classic labeling theory focuses solely on self-perception. It studies how one perceives himself when he is formally labeled and when he sees the difference in the way he is viewed by others, including those who label him and those who know the label that has been applied to him. It also studies how self-perception prompts change in self-identity, specifically, how one begins to accept a label, sees himself as labeled, and uses the label to feed on his own behavior.

Besides self-perception, however, there are third-party perception and collective perception, each of which may also play a significant role in the process of identity change. Third-party perception refers to views and feelings toward a label and a so-labeled person by his or her family members, relatives, friends, peers, co-workers, and neighbors. In the case of marijuana, if significant third parties do not take the label of marijuana grower, use, or user seriously, a person who is formally labeled by law enforcement as a violator in marijuana may not feel any shame from labeling or any pressure to change him or herself one way or the other. On the other hand, when significant third parties take a label, such as IV user or heroin addict, at its face value, a person who is so formally diagnosed and treated by medical authorities may feel he is indeed different from what he was before. Acting upon third-party perception about his serious reality as labeled, he may continue his slide toward helpless addiction or seek help to recover from it.

Collective perception is shared by people in a group, organization, community, culture, or society about a label and a subject or object so labeled. Labeling theory identifies perception as a critical variable because it is through perception that a labeled subject begins to change the way he or she views and behaves him or herself. Collective perception obviously does not exist inside a labeled subject. The way it acts upon the subject and his or her identity is therefore quite different. Specifically, when people know about a label and relate the label to a subject or object, they begin to see and approach the subject or object the way it is labeled. As it is powerful, collective perception usually prevails and persists even when the subject attempts to clear him or herself from the label. For instance, users who use less harmful drugs in a controlled manner may still be seen in collective perception as drug abusers who not only hurt themselves but also violate social norms. Similarly, substance use may still be equalized as drug abuse by collective perception even though in fact only a small portion of substance use falls under abuse. For a particular substance, once it is labeled as a dangerous drug leading to addiction on the basis of commonsense knowledge or preliminary evidence, people will view and treat it accordingly even later when scientific research proves it to be otherwise. Since substance and substance use as objects or things do not have their own "self-perception" to mediate between an imposing label and their "subsequent behavior," collective perception remains the only medium where the label assumes meaning and labeling takes effect.

Primary Substance Use

Primary substance use takes place before use is identified and the user is labeled. When substance use is examined per se, primary use may sound like a nonintentional, accidental, or excusable initial act. However, when the whole deviant career or labeling experience of a person is taken into account, primary substance use may in fact be a secondary deviation or act resulting from a formal labeling process. For instance, one is expelled from school and turns to substance use as he or she is known as a dropout; one joins a gang and uses drugs as he or she sees him- or herself as a formal gang member; and one is not successful in his or her conventional pursuits or in his or her unconventional endeavors. He or she engages in drug use when he or she retreats from active life as a loser.

Secondary Substance Use

Secondary substance use follows a formal labeling process in which users are recognized as specific types or classes of users and they begin to so perceive and behave themselves in their use and nonuse environments. Analogous to the case of primary substance use, secondary substance use may serve as primary acts or deviations for some users to acquire labels other than substance use and to take on identities other than substance users or abusers. For instance, a drinker operates a vehicle after a considerable intake of alcohol. He is stopped by the police and is treated as a law violator in the name of driving while under the influence of alcohol; a male user takes a drug himself and drugs his female counterpart to take sexual advantage of her. He is charged with rape and is viewed as a rapist; and a street drug user engages in a violent robbery to obtain money for his or her addictive habit. He or she is caught by the law enforcement agency and is punished as a criminal.

Obviously, substance use may be linked to various other life events in a user's whole experience. Labeling, delabeling, and relabeling may take place in a continuing process as users enter into and exit from different activities and roles amid their substance use.

Theoretical Applications

The central question raised by the social reaction perspective is: what role and how significantly does social reaction play in the initiation, escalation, habituation, or termination of an individual's substance use? Various specific questions or theoretical applications can be explored under this central theme.

Regarding social reaction, while sanctions imposed by legal and moral authorities, such as the government and church, remain most binding and forceful, a wide range of social entities or influences may serve to initiate, reinforce, or sustain negative, neutral, or positive labeling for different substances, substance uses, and substance users. Specifically, how do general attitudes toward substance use in a society play out in the labeling process? How does collective perception about substance use in a culture influence label assigners and bearers in their attitudes and behaviors? How does third-party perception about substance use in a user's surroundings affect the user's acceptance of a labeled identity? Also, how do formal authorities fight or cooperate with informal social sources in labeling and treating substance use and users? For instance, while the government explicitly condemns drug users as politically defying or morally decaying rebels or addicts, the mass media, liberal critics, and the entertainment industry may implicitly glamorize substance users as innovative or courageous adventurers or revolutionaries.

With respect to users, the social reaction perspective is not just fixated on the passive part of their being label bearers. It also raises questions about the active role of their being actors who initiate, reflect upon, and attempt to conform to or rebel against social responses. First, why do they engage in substance use? Is it because they are labeled in other domains as dropouts, troublemakers, delinquents, or losers? Or is it because they want to gain attention, earn a reputation in something, and bear a label, positive or negative, just to be different? Second, when they are labeled as substance users or into different statuses of use, how do they perceive their acquired labels as well as their changed reality so that they feel comfortable with what they are or motivated to move forward to what they want to be? No matter what pressure they may receive from their surroundings in the labeling process, it is in the end the users who decide what course of action to take in their own reaction. In an open society where the label of substance use or abuse is not as devastating as criminality to one's positive identity, why do a lot of users still seem to be so ready to take on new user identities in their progressive substance use career? Does labeling really matter? Or is it just secondary compared to the addictive nature of a substance used and the psychological and physiological dependence gradually developed by the user? Third, once they internalize a user label, do users stabilize in the state designated by the label? Or do they use it as a springboard to jump into a higher state of use and problem behavior for yet another labeling process? Specifically, what does it take to make one a self-sufficient habitual user—a stable supply, a tolerant social network, or noninterference from law enforcement? Or what goes wrong when one escalates from mild to severe user status and ends up dead in an emergency room? Is an intolerant public, a penetrative law enforcement, or a generally punitive social reaction to blame?

As far as substances and substance use are concerned, the fact that they are classified into different categories and given labels of different meanings makes them qualify for study in light of the social reaction perspective. A substance is an object. It itself does not have any self-consciousness to perceive a label assigned to it nor to change what it is in subsequent interactions with human subjects. However, as it is labeled by human subjects, it will subsequently receive different evaluations and treatments from them. In theoretical applications, it is therefore meaningful to explore how a label is first assigned to a substance or a type of substance use: is the label based upon age-old perception, commonsense knowledge, media misinformation, subculture lingo, or hearsay? Why is a substance or a form of use stuck with a label once it is given the label? What specific forces, historical, political, economic, cultural, or social, are there to keep a label to the substance or the form of use so labeled? How does a label guide users as well as people in the general public to fantasize, chase, indulge in, glamorize, fear, distance from, evilize, or hate a substance or a type of use? And what does it take to unravel the mystery of a label and to liberate a substance or a form of use from its long-held label—scientific evidence, change of law, or change of time?

At the macro level, a society, a generation, or an era may be made known or labeled as having a high or low level of use of one or multiple substances. Society, generation, or era is both object and subject. It is object because it is not as self-conscious as a human subject. When it is labeled as having certain attributes, it does not directly take on those attributes and act accordingly. It is subject because it includes self-conscious human subjects within itself. When it is known for certain characteristics, people who live in it may perceive themselves sharing those characteristics and hence so synchronize their thoughts and behaviors. The dual, objective and subjective nature of social and historical systems obviously opens a barrage of questions for theoretical exploration. On the objective side, why and how does a society, generation, or era become known for substance use? Is it due to impressions by sojourners, reports by mass media, or research by scientists? Is it grounded in statistics compiled by the government, stories written by novelists, or cases gathered by clinicians? On the subjective side, how is a reputation for a society, generation, or era spread among people who live within it? How is it perceived by those who share the reputation? To what extent does it affect individuals in their thoughts and acts? As any particular individual may be either aware or unaware of, relevant or irrelevant to, and receptive or resistant to a reputation he or she shares with others in his or her society, generation, or era, what ultimate consequence does a label have for the so-labeled society, generation, or era? Does the label necessarily reinforce the primary acts that lead to the society, generation, or historical era being labeled in the first place? What secondary acts will it result in?

Empirical Tests

To answer various theoretical questions derived from the social reaction perspective, specific empirical studies need to be conducted using different research methods.

Case studies are appropriate for both users and substances. The value of a case may lie in its typicality, uniqueness, or the fact that it can be studied in great detail. Typical cases may include a user who is initially labeled due to other actions than drug use, who labels him or herself in order to fit in a crowd, who takes great pride in bearing a particular user label, who is devastated by a stigmatizing label, who has never been formally labeled but proceeds persistently in his or her substance use career, who fights vehemently against a label toward successful delabeling, or who has been through a full circle of labeling, delabeling, and relabeling in his or her use and treatment experience. The focus of research may be put on either the general process, from labeling to inner reaction to identity change to subsequent behavior, or specific issues in the process, such as pressure from the environment, damage on self-image, and identity-prompted behavioral adjustment. Since the number of substances used and abused is not as large as the number of users, each substance can be studied as an individual case. Specifically, it is insightful to detail what labels a particular substance is given by the authority, the public, and its users; how a given label defines and influences the general impression, perception, and attitude each of those three sources holds toward the substance; what it takes for a substance to break away from a label for a new image in society; and how much each of those factors, including natural properties, age-old knowledge, scientific evidence, and use subculture of or about a substance, weighs in the social labeling, delabeling, and relabeling process for the substance.

Historical analysis may combine with case studies to follow some typical users in their whole labeling experience: how they are first labeled, how labeling in one area of their life leads to labeling in the other, how labeling in substance use proceeds in terms of severity or status, how labeling takes place in response to escalation, treatment, recovery, and abstinence, and how labeling is related to change in perception, identity, and behavior. Most important, historical analysis is essential to cataloging names, labels, and their respective meanings given to a substance over time as well as to understanding a particular reputation in substance use earned by a society in a specific generation or era. For instance, why is a substance initially named X? Why does it take on other names in addition to or in replacement of X later in its existence? How does each of its names affect its perception and use by the public? Similarly, how is a particular reputation for substance use developed in a society? Is it due to environmental factors, evolutionary adaptation, war, trade, religious movement, political change, or cultural intrusion? How is the reputation passed on from generation to generation, through childhood socialization, rites of passage to adulthood, or other institutional practices? How does it fade from history? Or how does one reputation give rise to another across generations or a historical era?

Interview and survey research provide suitable tools to study what labelers intend in creating and assigning a label for substance, use, or user; how people generally react to the label; and, most important, how labelees interpret the label, deal with label-prompted reactions from their surroundings, take on a new identity as labeled, and act in accordance with changes in their own perception and identity. While observation from the outside of a subject helps detect attitudinal and behavioral changes, it is interview and survey research that explore the inner world of the subject, revealing the real and moment-to-moment connections between perception and behavior. For instance, when observation shows an increase of use in the aftermath of labeling, only interview can find out whether labeling acts upon the subject positively, negatively, or neutrally. In other words, only the subject can tell whether he or she takes pride in a label, becoming motivated to enhance his or her newly obtained fame with more use, or labeling takes a negative toll, pushing him or her further into severe use.

Experimental studies are useful in comparing effects of labels and labeling for or on substances, substance use, and users. For example, a substance may be given no label, a label as a controlled drug, and a label as a nutritional supplement for three groups of comparable subjects to dispose of in a period of three weeks or to just think of all possible use reactions they may have in a one-hour session. Results can be insightful to the issue of how labels given to a substance shape public attitudes toward the substance. Similarly, drug users admitted to a treatment center may be divided into three comparable groups. Each group is informed by a seemingly authoritative figure of a specific diagnosis: no dependency, mild dependency, or severe dependency. It is then given the opportunity to choose different regimens of treatment available at the center. Outcomes from the experiment may shed light on the relationship between labeling and behavioral adaptation. It is obvious that various experimental studies can be creatively and innovatively designed to examine differences and similarities between labeling and nonlabeling, between positive labeling and negative labeling, among different labels, and along progressively negative or positive labels in application to substances, forms of use, and types of users.

POLICY IMPLICATIONS

The social reaction perspective is a self-reflective approach on social reaction itself. Substances become known and available. Substance use takes place. Substance users make onset to, proceed with, and maturate from use. All these cause social reactions. However, social reactions, while purporting to reduce, halt, or eliminate substance use, may actually play an important part in making it a continuing, expanding, or exacerbating social problem. The often inevitable unintended consequence presents agents and agencies in social reaction arenas with tremendous challenges.

Public Health

Prevention begins with a clear identification of risk behaviors and risk-taking individuals. When a risk behavior is marked for prevention, it may solidify as an act of courage, bravery, rebellion, or other worth in the eyes of risk takers, calling for more effort from prevention. When a risk taker is identified, he or she may take on the identity and act not only accordingly but also in a more outstanding manner. Prevention hence becomes self-perpetuating: it makes itself more necessary and more urgent. In other words, once there is a prevention team in place, sooner or later there will be a need for a larger team to conduct a seemingly increased task.

Medical intervention requires an accurate diagnosis of symptoms. When a symptom is determined to result from the intake of a substance, it may be externalized as a material condition by the symptom bearer: "It is caused by that substance. I have no control over it." When a substance user of a specific syndrome is identified as a drug addict or dependent user, he or she may use the diagnosis as an excuse to retreat from productive life into the world of the so-diagnosed identity: "I am a drug addict. I have long lost control over that substance. What am I supposed to do now in relation to the substance?" Similar to prevention, medical intervention can harden its target and make itself a continuing or ever-challenging pursuit for its own sake.

With recognition of the possible countereffect of their respective effort, prevention and medical intervention can improve themselves in the following key aspects. First, problem identification, symptom diagnosis, and label assignment should be strictly based upon facts and scientific evidence. Second, labels and terms used for risks and medical conditions should be checked for and cleared from any of their possible moral connotations and political overtures. Third, the atmosphere for prevention and environment in medical treatment should be humanized to accommodate needs by targeted subjects and treated patients rather than to alienate them for their problem experiences. Fourth, care and reservation should be exercised by prevention and medical professionals in creating, assigning, and communicating risks, diagnoses, and labels to targeted subjects and treated patients, especially given their inherent temptation or tendency to overlabel problems and symptoms in practice. Fifth, risk identification, medical diagnosis, or labeling in general should be synchronized with subjects' or patients' inner feelings and perceptions to motivate them to objectively admit, positively face, and actively fight their risks or medical conditions amid the professional support and treatment received from the outside.

Social Control

Agents and agencies in social control are normally programmed to act on their targets with certainty, swiftness, and severity. Although their actions are charged with a high level of moral input, they usually do not reserve much time to reflect upon what consequences their actions bring about in the minds of their targeted subjects. It may sound plainly absurd to them that they and their actions play a role in making a correctable habit an incurable disease, a minor infraction a serious violation, a recreational drug user a helpless addict, or a novice offender a career criminal.

While the social reaction perspective does not intend to prevent social control agents from taking any action at all against substance use, it provides them with useful warnings so that they can minimize possible negative repercussions when they approach the issue. First, labeling certain substances as illicit or controlled substances may have inadvertently made them hardened targets in social control. When the classification system is torn down, all substances can be treated equally in terms of their actual use by and consequence for users and society. Second, defining certain substance uses as legal violations may have overextended the reach of social control into the area of substance use. When use itself is not legalized or illegalized by a social authority, individual discretion will naturally step in as an often more effective form of social control. Third, casting certain substance users as addicts or law violators may have virtually motivated them in their expectations for and dependence upon social intervention. When substance users are cleared from legal and moral complications, they can be more effectively treated for whatever health problems they may have toward recovery. In general, current social control reactions toward substance use may indeed have made things worse or more difficult to control. To minimize possible negative repercussions, agents and agencies in social control should leave the large chunk of the issue to science, individual discretion, and medicine and react only when substance users have committed crimes against the person or property by way of use or in the aftermath of abuse.

Life and Community

Community serves as a critical medium by which a label is transmitted from its imposing authority to the imposed individual. It affects how the label is interpreted by the people relevant to the individual and hence how it is eventually perceived by the individual.

With the social reaction perspective in sight, people in the community can be cautioned to act in a way that makes the community a buffering zone rather than a facilitating context to labeling and its negative effect. First, they remain open-minded to and tolerant of different lifestyles in their community so that they do not automatically and impulsively single out a particular habit, substance use, or user as a nuisance or troublemaker. Second, they face specific incidents or situations in their life so that they do not naturally and simplistically generalize particular episodes, substance uses, or users into a general kind of events or people in their reference system. For instance, when one of their neighbors gets drunk frequently or occasionally, they specifically state that he or she becomes drunk there and then, but do not abstractly charge that he or she is a drunkard, an alcoholic, or an irresponsible person. Similarly, instead of calling someone a marijuana user, a smoker, or an addict, they objectively state that he or she uses marijuana, smokes cigarettes, or has problems with drugs. Third, they maintain a critical mind so that they are always suspicious of labels placed on individuals in their surroundings by the authorities or from the outside. For example, the effect of labeling can be totally blocked out when no one in the community follows the authority in labeling and treating a marijuana grower or user as a law violator. Fourth, they have a sympathetic, accommodating, and supportive heart so that they readily and warmly welcome and accept as their dear relatives and neighbors those who were once labeled substance users, drug addicts, deviants, or criminal offenders. Delabeling, relabeling, rebirth, and return to the mainstream life can therefore be expedited, smoothened, and solidified.

Work and Organization

Although workplaces do not tend to serve as sites where substance users are formally labeled, work and organizations may still directly or indirectly influence how substance use is initiated, why labeling in substance use takes place, and whether delabeling from substance use is successful.

First, work is a potential source of stress. Work organizations are poised to label people as reliable or unreliable performers, conscientious or untrustworthy employees, and low or high achievers. Rewards and penalties are well instituted to reinforce labels and labeling processes as basic organizational routines or rhetoric. Striving for rewards and positive labels may motivate people to use performance-enhancing substances, such as steroids and other drugs used by athletes. Being labeled as underachievers, suspended from active duty, or laid off from work may drive people into a situation where they turn to substance use as a means of relief, a way of escape, or a symbol of rebellion.

Second, organization provides an authoritative context where labels are created, ascertained, assigned, interpreted, and made effective by and onto individuals. A person who is known as a recreational drug user in his community may not take that externally given status seriously in his life settings. But if he is identified as a drug-impaired employee by his employment organization, he may really mix that verdict with his internal feelings and thoughts about work, self-image, and self-identity. In a broader sense, organizations include governmental agencies, social services, substance use treatment facilities, clinics, hospitals, universities, and research centers where labeling originates, becomes clarified and sanctified, and ends. For instance, various labels circulated by users in the street surface with definite meanings in mainstream language and communications only when reporters and scholars in media and research organizations have dug them out, verified them, and properly framed them for general presentation.

Third, work may serve as reward toward recovery while organizations may offer collective support for quitting substance users. In drug abuse treatment programs, former patients work as counselors and role models. The fact that they work as self-sufficient members of society not only reinforces their own delabeling process from chemical dependency, but also encourages their help-seeking clients to overcome use identity toward relabeling and rebirth. In a larger social context, working with a source of income is the most important indicator that a drug addict or criminal has successfully delabeled him- or herself from his or her former deviant identity. Being employed in an organization represents the most important symbol of recognition that a former substance abuser or social cast has been fully relabeled by the society as one of its productive members.

Recognizing the stake of work and organization in the construction, perpetuation, and deconstruction of positive and negative labels pertaining to substance use, deviance, and criminality, employers, employees, and other organizational stakeholders should not only take basic precautions to avoid exacerbating an already bad situation, but also take necessary actions to reinforce every sign of promise in the case of positive development.

In all, the social reaction perspective alerts all social authorities about the possible negative effect of their respectively perceived positive reactions to substances, substance use, and substance users. Social authorities range from families, schools, community organizations, employers, medical establishments, social service agencies, and cultural institutions, to the criminal justice system. The self-perceived positive actions they usually take toward substance use and users include diagnosis, prevention, treatment, disciplining, expulsion, condemnation, shaming, and incarceration. The possible negative effects from such punitive or stigmatizing actions vary from substance to substance, user to user, society to society, generation to generation, and era to era. For example, a substance being controlled as an illicit drug may draw serious interest from various social groups, expanding its use more widely across the population. A user being diagnosed by the medical establishment as a drug addict or being punished by the criminal justice system as a drug law offender may take on the identity as diagnosed or treated, deviating further away from recovery and the mainstream. A society, generation, or historical era engulfed by a drug war may emerge with a vengeance of epidemic use of a multitude of substances, becoming a more hardened target for drug war onslaughts.

Should there be no social reactions at all given the complicating effects of social reactions on substance use and users? While the social reaction perspective is primarily interested in revealing and studying the effects of social reactions, implications for policy and practice are quite obvious. In a nutshell, agents and agencies in social reactions should not spend all their time and energy on labeling substances, chasing substance users, and blaming a morally decaying generation or society for rampant substance use and abuse. Instead, they should keep some time and space to reflect upon the way they set up rules, educate the young, define deviance and crimes, approach substance use, and treat substance users. In some situations, the best way to react to substance use is to take no action at all. In some situations, the less action taken, the better it is for substance use and users. But under all circumstances, users and uses themselves should first be given their full respective force or right in correcting, healing, or adjusting a temporarily problematic situation before any social reaction ever takes place.

—10—

The Subculture Perspective

Society is a gathering place. People aggregate around similarities in background, identity, belief, value, interest, and practice. Substance use, as an act or practice embodying specific beliefs and values, can obviously bring people together to form distinctive groupings and subcultures, different from other subculture collectives or the mainstream social system.

The subculture perspective focuses on the inner workings of substance user groups and groupings. It examines what beliefs, values, norms, and rituals users develop and follow in preserving and sustaining their substance use. It inspects what props, tools, aids, and equipment users innovate and employ in preparing substances for use, in administering substances, or in sanctifying use itself. It explores why users come together and what keeps them in solidarity with each other in the process of use, in the aftermath of abuse, as well as in reaction to pressure from the outside. Noting the variety of subcultures adjacent to substance use, the subculture perspective also attends to substance-related subcultures, such as the youth subculture, prostitute subculture, gang subculture, and deviant subculture, to see how each of those neighboring subcultures relates to substance use as cause, collateral occurrence, or consequence.

SOURCES OF INSPIRATION

Work by Frederic Thrasher and William Whyte represents some of the earliest writings on subcultures. Thrasher (1927) developed a typology to describe different types of gangs he studied in Chicago. Drawing upon Thrasher, Whyte (1943) further advanced the subcultural thesis through his research on the Italian slum he called "Cornerville." Whyte found that lower-class slum residents can achieve success through such opportunities as racketeering and bookmaking, afforded by the slum culture.

Albert Cohen (1955), a student of Edwin Sutherland as well as ot Robert Merton, provides a full account of how the delinquent subculture arises and where it is located within the larger social structure by combining Sutherland's notion of deviance learning with Merton's theory of social strain. According to Cohen, American youths from all backgrounds are generally held accountable to the norms of the wider society, or what he called "the middle-class measuring rod." The measures are based on such middle-class values as self-reliance, cleanliness, neatness, punctuality, respect for property, long-range planning, proficiency in language, competency in school performance, and competitiveness in job duty. Lower-class children obviously face great disadvantage by these measures as they grow up with poor communication skills, lack of commitment to education, and an inability to delay gratification in families that have never known a middle-class lifestyle. In response to status frustration and strain they experience from competitions with middle-class children in school and on other fronts, they usually adopt one of three roles: corner boy, college boy, or delinquent boy. Corner boys hang out in the neighborhood. They participate in group activities, such as gambling, games, and athletic competitions, and maintain effective bonds with one another. College boys strive to live up middle-class standards despite many of their academic and social handicaps. Delinquent boys join hands to form a subculture by which they overcome their loss of self-esteem, improve their sense of self-worth, and achieve status. They may destroy what they have stolen or engage in vandalism and other nonutilitarian delinquencies just to expressly fire off their hostility toward middle-class values. Cohen views such delinquent behavior as a result of middle-class values turned upside down. Borrowing from psychoanalysis, he terms it reaction formation, "the process in which a person openly rejects that which he wants, or aspires to, but cannot obtain or achieve" (Shoemaker 1984: 102).

Richard Cloward and Lloyd Ohlin (1960) offer a different picture of delinquent subcultures in their joint work on delinquency and opportunity. Like Cohen, they combine strain, differential association, and social disorganization concepts in their theory building. Unlike Cohen, however, they realize that delinquent subcultures are not necessarily in square opposition to what is espoused in the dominant culture. Instead, they point out that just as means to reach one's goals are unequally distributed in the conventional world, opportunities are not equally and readily available to everyone who wants to pursue an unconventional career. In areas where deviant values gain currency and illegitimate businesses take root, youths join criminal networks and learn proper techniques, motives, and connections from adult criminals. Criminal gangs emerge. A criminal subculture forms to support and sustain crime as a means toward profit and material success. In neighborhoods of transience and instability where neither criminal nor conventional adult role models exist for emulation, youngsters engage in fighting and destructive violence to deal with boredom and tiredness, to release anger and anxiety, or to demonstrate courage and toughness. Conflict gangs flourish. A conflict subculture arises to justify and legitimize violence as a means to gain status. The third type is a retreatist subculture. It provides fertile soil for the formation and operation of retreatist gangs among those who fail not only in the conventional world, but also in their attempt to join in organized criminal activity and violence-oriented gangs. Retreatists withdraw from a productive lifestyle and hide in a world of drunkenness, addiction, dependency, vagrancy, or homelessness. According to Cloward and Ohlin (1960), delinquent subcultures have at least three identifiable features: "(a) acts of delinquency that reflect subcultural support are likely to recur with great frequency, (b) access to a successful adult criminal career sometimes results from participation in a delinquent subculture, and (c) the delinquent subculture imparts to the conduct of its members a high degree of stability and resistance to control or change" (12–13).

Focusing on violence, Marvin Wolfgang and Franco Ferracuti (1967) identify a subculture of violence that exists in some lower-class urban communities. To many young males who are born and raised in the subculture, violence is a way of life. They grow up amid violence, from being spanked by parents, witnessing one parent being battered by the other, and participating in street gang warfare, to being drawn into some kind of collective brawls. They carry knives, clubs, or guns not only as weapons of protection, but also as tools of aggression. They use fists rather than words to settle disputes. They feel no sense of guilt or regret toward whoever triumphs or falls in violence, including themselves. Since violence is inherently integrated in the subcultural value system, nonviolence and people who do not resort to violence may even be condemned and reprimanded. The subculture of violence can persist through associational learning from one age group to another. In fact, once it is established in a community, it may survive for generations before it possibly fades away completely.

While the subculture of violence seems to suggest that deviant subcultures grow and develop on their own terms, it is Walter Miller (1958) who first looks into the lower-class culture itself in his study of juvenile gangs. Different from Cohen, Cloward, and Ohlin, who conceptualize delinquent subcultures as manifest rejections of middle-class values, Miller argues that gang norms are simply the adolescent expression of the lower-class culture that, apart from the middle-class culture, exists and evolves for generations in disadvantaged neighborhoods. According to Miller, there are six focal concerns among youths who grow up in lower-class environments. First is concern over trouble. Trouble may range from fighting, drinking, and sexual misbehaving, to an encounter with the law. As daily preoccupation, youth need to constantly stay in or out of trouble so that they can command the most prestige among peers. Second is concern over toughness. To the large proportion of lower-class males who come from female-dominated households, masculinity, physical strength, and rejection of sentimentality are the most favorable personal qualities to have and to show off. Joining street gangs represents an easy or only avenue by which they find male role models with whom they can identify. Third is concern over smartness. Outsmarting others is favored and actively pursued by youth in games, exchanges, and other daily activities. Youths gain respect when they demonstrate smartness. Fourth is concern over excitement. Facing a high level of boredom and tiredness in daily life, lower-class youth seek excitement by hanging out with peers and by taking risks, such as drug abuse and car racing. Fifth is concern over luck. Feeling a sense of lack of control over their fate, youth place hope for a quick change in life on lotteries, cards, dice, and other gambles. The last concern is over autonomy. In response to an excessive degree of control they often receive from parents, teachers, and the police, youth desire personal freedom and resent external manipulations. From time to time, they proclaim to both themselves and others: "No one can push me around" and "I do not need nobody."

The idea that a background or home culture provides primary sources of inspiration and support for a delinquent subculture that grows within its soil opens up research on gangs and delinquency in major population groups or social contexts. Research on female gangs examines the female culture in an attempt to explain why some female gangs become male affiliates, why some become independent, and how girls, similar to or different from boys, join gangs for mutual support, protection, and a sense of belonging (Campbell 1984). Studies on middle-class delinquency and suburban gangs focus on middle-class values in their efforts to explain why delinquent gangs, hate gangs, and satanic gangs arise in the context of middle-class living and thinking (Korem 1994). Investigations of contemporary gangs overall explore the large cultural environment to fathom why guns and weapons proliferate in gang warfare and why gangs increasingly engage in turf battles surrounding drug trafficking, gambling, prostitution, and other profitable businesses (Fagan 1993; Blumstein 1995).

Centering on the youth culture that is believed to provide contextual support for juvenile delinquency, a whole research tradition has come into existence in describing and analyzing adolescents with respect to their own cultural sources and resources. Ernest Smith (1962) points out that contemporary society provides no clearly defined status roles for youth, except the dependent-subordinate roles of children and students, which often alienate them as they begin to view themselves as young adults. Hans Sebald (1968) identifies five key elements that together make the youth subculture differ from the mainstream culture. The five key elements of the youth subculture include: common values and norms, different from those of adults and those for children; unique lingo and argots, not necessarily understood and approved by adults; common styles and fads, evident in hairstyles, tattoos, dressing, grooming, and makeup; distinctive forms of mass media, represented by magazines, movies, music, and television programs with appeal to youths; and distinctive criteria for status, as illustrated by what adolescents look up to in their peers, leaders, and role models. According to Sebald, the youth subculture serves youth three major purposes: a sense of belonging, gratification of specific needs, and social support. All these functions are crucially important to youths as they look to peers for answers and solutions in dealing with the marginality they suffer from in family and school as well as the uncertainty they face in the larger social structure (Schwendinger and Schwendinger 1985; Begley 2000).

As far as substance use is concerned, studies using the concept or perspective of subculture divide into two major groups. The first group examines various subcultures, including racial, ethnic, gay and lesbian, homeless, criminal, college student, blue-collar worker, athlete, professional, street, and regional, to see how each of them encourages or discourages substance use. For instance, between the youth subculture and substance use, rebellion against parents, loyalty to peers, and risk as challenge are found to be the core values and motives behind adolescent drug use (Glassner and Loughlin 1987; Jones and Bell-Bolek 1986; McGee 1992). As Evan Thomas (1986) succinctly points out, "in the age of youth rebellion, the fact that parents were shocked by drugs was all the more reason for children to take them." Between the industrial subculture and substance use, Craig Janes and Genevieve Ames (1989) conducted research on white assembly-line workers in a large durable-goods manufacturing plant in California. They found that heavy drinking is supported and sustained by a workplace subculture featuring the boredom of repetitive blue-collar work, job frustration, and lack of outside social alternatives. As drinking serves as a crucial way of improving interpersonal communication and social relationships, only a few of those who become involved in community and social activities with their families and friends, excluding their co-workers, are able to resist the workplace subculture to stay free from alcohol.

The second group of studies delve into the drug subculture and many of its subsidiaries, from narcotic subculture, wine subculture, intravenous use subculture, international drug subculture, and drug dealer/seller subculture, to drug abstinent subculture, to learn what rule and attitude are developed, what skill and technique are spread, and what strategy and tactic are adopted. Edmundo Morales (1986) compared the marketing aspect of the international drug subcultures concerning coca paste, bazuco, and chicle in Peru and crack cocaine in the United States. Samuel

Friedman and Cathy Casriel (1988) investigated the intravenous drug use subculture in their effort to understand why intravenous drug users have failed to develop self-organization as gay males for the provision of health care, education, and support. Natti Ronel (1998) followed Narcotics Anonymous as a subculture of recovery that bridges the drug subculture and the prevailing culture. Inherent in the so-conceived subculture of recovery are the following essential components: sobriety as an innovation, recovery as a basis for value systems and behavioral norms, the language and rituals of recovery, and social situations, role definitions, and actions related to recovery. On the drug culture as a whole, Victor Shaw (1999) provides a comprehensive analysis with respect to its variety, underlying force, and user function. According to him, "drug culture varies by community, type of drug, race, language, and social class it is shaped by two basic forces: (a) the need for group recognition and collective justification for drug use as a socially stigmatized behavior, and (b) the need for protection against law enforcement officials, who view drug use as an illegal behavior" (35). For users in particular, "drug culture enables users to develop drug-obtaining networks and resources; share drug-using devices, techniques, rituals, and feelings; participate in activities prompted by drug effects, and cope with problems associated with drug use" (35).

THEORETICAL FRAMEWORK

The subculture perspective implies that substance use is a collective behavior. It begins with a segment of the population who share beliefs and values in favor of certain substances and their consumption. It sustains among the collective whose members come together to mutually provide both ideological justification and material support for their common habit. It evolves along with the general social climate as well as the specific subculture in which it occurs.

Definition

Culture is the total way of life in a society. Among the innumerable aspects of life are two major components of culture. One is spiritual or nonmaterial culture, which includes beliefs, values, norms, feelings, and sentiments. The other is behavioral or material culture, which includes acts, deeds, arts, crafts, constructions, creations, and other material achievements, such as houses, farms, irrigation networks, automobiles, factories, cities, and ballistic missiles. Culture is shared and learned. It spreads from individual to individual, group to group, generation to generation, and society to society.

Subculture is a shared way of life among a group of people in a society. On the one hand, subculture builds upon the general culture. It constitutes the general culture. It enriches the general culture. On the other hand, it differs from the general culture. It challenges the general culture. It may even rebel against the general culture. Among various subcultures that come into existence in contemporary society, there are urban, suburban, and rural subcultures; professional, craftsman, and manual labor subcultures; conventional, deviant, and criminal subcultures; or upper-, middle-, and lower-class subcultures. According to Erich Goode (1994), members of a group that subscribes to a particular subculture interact with one another more frequently and more intimately than they do with members of other social categories; have a way of life and beliefs that are somewhat different from those of members of other social categories; and think of themselves as belonging to a specific group.

The drug or substance subculture is a subculture shared by substance users regarding substance supply, preparation, use, problem solving, user interactions, and user-society relations. To users, it provides essential motives and techniques required in the process of substance use. To nonusers, it offers critical explanations and justifications as to why substance use is necessary, inevitable, beneficial, or nonharmful. Inside the substance subculture, it may vary in content or form by the substance used, the procedure adopted, the tool employed, and the user involved. For instance, there specifically might be a marijuana subculture, an alcohol subculture, an intravenous drug use subculture, a chewing tobacco subculture, or a professional drug user subculture. At the outset, the substance subculture may lie within the general culture of a society. It may also go beyond individual societies to become a universal culture of its own across a country, a continent, a civilization, and even the whole world. As a result, it is legitimate and meaningful to talk about the coca culture in South America, the wine and beer culture in Western civilizations, and the substance use and abuse culture on the face of the earth.

The subculture perspective is a theoretical exploration into the body of the substance subculture. It examines all the structural elements and their interrelations within the substance subculture. It follows the change and evolution of the substance culture through groups of users as well as over generations of users. It investigates various functions the substance subculture serves for users and nonusers. It also looks into ways the substance subculture contributes to or counteracts the dominant mainstream culture.

Theoretical Image

The subculture perspective provides a unique imagery of how substance, substance use, and substance users each originate from or give rise to, as well as persist or survive in, social groupings or collective environments.

Substance can serve as a material base for a subculture to grow and thrive. In the subculture surrounding a particular substance or a group of them, whether it is tobacco, alcohol, prescription drugs, or controlled substances, there are public attitudes, legal statutes, legends, folklore, and statistical records about it. There is general knowledge regarding its properties, its physical and chemical forms, and its medicinal, therapeutic, or poisonous values. There are specific techniques on how to grow, gather, synthesize, produce, process, store, transport, and market it. There are directions, warnings, and advice on the preparation of the substance for use, the proper procedure of consumption, and the management of the symptoms following its use. There are medical, group, and social reactions to or treatment for the substance-related problems or consequences. There is hardware, from farm, factory, and equipment, to packaging materials, specially made for the production of the substance. There is labor power, including growers, potters, chemists, and doctors, specially trained for the handling of the substance. All these subcultural elements pertaining to a substance combine to make the substance an enduring feature in a society throughout a period of time, or even over the whole human life. For instance, both the alcohol and the tobacco subcultures have followed human civilizations for an unmeasurably long time. Each now involves a whole operation across industry, commerce, service, medicine, and even justice.

Substance use can act as a domain for a subculture to form and expand. While use is often specific to individual substances, it can rise above various substance-specific use situations, serving as a common ground for the formation of a general use subculture. A general substance use subculture may feature a fundamental belief in the power of substance. For instance, members of the subculture believe that substance is the ultimate element or force to create, correct, or eliminate certain conditions within human beings. The subculture may place great emphasis on the process of use. For example, members of the subculture make serious efforts to create and administer protocols, rituals, or ceremonies as necessary and inevitable elements of use and use procedure. A general use subculture may also highlight use as art, craft, entertainment, adventure, protest, rebellion, mental escape, spiritual emancipation, status, or lifestyle. In that regard, members of the subculture may share their peculiar feelings, moods, sentiments, or journeys, through writing or club-based interactions, from certain unique ways of use of one substance or a combination of substances.

Substance users are drawn into a substance when they are exposed to a subculture pertaining to the substance. Established users constitute the core of the substance use subculture. Within it, they maintain, expand, and update use-related knowledge, technology, skills, beliefs, norms, values, rituals, justifications, and rationalizations. They invent, guard, and employ specific tools, procedures, and facilities. They sponsor and participate in activities that embody the spirit of use. They share and exchange concerns, secrets, feelings, and sentiments. They deal with physical, psychological, and medical problems resulting from use. They coordinate reactions to law enforcement intervention and social criticism. They take initiatives to transmit appropriate knowledge and beliefs to new, young, and inexperienced users. To the outside, members of the substance use subculture network with their relatives, friends, neighbors, coworkers, peers, and further with the general public. They not only influence them in their attitudes toward substance, substance use, and substance users, but also attract or drag them to the substance subculture as observer, sympathizer, or potential entrant. They may even reach out to the legal, medical, academic, and other professional communities, in various forms of media presentation, to win sympathy and support from different social sectors or to neutralize the general negative view held by the populace about substance use and abuse.

Spatially, the substance subculture draws upon and contributes to other subcultures as well as the general culture in critical inputs, important references, and general support. Critical inputs may include both software and hardware, such as knowledge, techniques, terms, motives, strategies, devices, and equipment. For instance, the substance subculture learns from deviant and criminal subcultures about strategies and tactics against criminal justice interventions. It borrows from scientific and medical subcultures specific methods of substance preparation, drug administration, and drug effect management. Important references give the substance subculture a comparative perspective with respect to its nature, scale, position, and social significance. General support stems from collective presence or action with other subcultures of similar causes or interests. For instance, a subculture of beauty and fitness may lend support, implicitly or explicitly, to a subculture of so-called health foods or nutritional supplements. A subculture of deviance or of a more negative nature may give manifest or latent reasons for the existence of a subculture of substance or of a lesser negative nature. Also, the substance subculture may align with other subcultures to ward off a common threat or attack from the conservative quarter, the mainstream, or some enemy subcultures in society. In the contemporary world, following trade, tourism, educational exchange, and multinational corporate expansion through advanced means of transportation and communication, the substance subculture is gradually breaking and may eventually tear down language, geographic, and other human barriers, becoming a subculture of its own across the globe. From Europe to North America, from the Equator to the North Pole, and from the cruise ships on the sea to the airliners in the sky, substance users share many aspects of their substance use despite the apparent differences in their skin colors, dress, tongues, and passports.

In history, the substance subculture follows human evolution and takes on specific features at each of its peculiar stages. In the very beginning, people search for, protect, and worship substances that show the mighty power of nature or the great deed of God. In the time of war, people look for, garner, and make substances they can use to kill the enemy, to cure wounds, or to boost the morale of soldiers. In the time of philosophical contemplation, people identify, prepare, and take substances they hope will enhance intelligence, broaden imagination, or alter human perception of the world. In the era of industrial production, people grow, synthesize, and administer substances they believe to have an impact on performance, appearance, and mood, or to have an effect on stress, pain, or hazardous environments they so often have to deal with. Across all different periods of time, people always experiment with substances to find beneficial, effective foods, medicines, poisons, and various special-purpose drugs to meet their ever-increasing practical needs in life. They also never stop searching for substances to satisfy their curiosity for, fantasy, or obsession with miracle, superpower, the extraordinary, the spiritual, or the transcendental. Entering the modern and postmodern era, material affluence, in all its conspicuousness, not only affirms people in their belief in the power of substance, but also empowers people in their disposal of substance. The substance subculture takes root deep and strong in the general culture as people take it for granted to use omnipresently available substances to enliven, enrich, and enhance their substance-based life.

Theoretical Components

The subculture perspective examines the substance subculture with regard to its internal structure and external relations. Inside, the substance subculture contains both material and nonmaterial elements. Outside, it engages in substantive exchange and interaction with other subcultures and the general culture.

Material Elements

In its material aspect, the substance subculture builds upon visible objects. First, there are primary substances, such as alcohol, tobacco, marijuana, and heroin. A substance, such as tea or cocaine, may come in different colors, packages, physical or chemical forms, quantities, qualities, and names. Some of its forms may be more pure, potent, or pricy than others. Second, there are raw materials that are used to make the substance and supplements that are used to accompany the substance during preparation or consumption. For instance, barley is grown to brew beer. Chemicals are used to synthesize methamphetamine. Milk and sugar are added to make coffee taste soft and sweet. Third, there are farms to grow raw materials, factories to manufacture the substance, laboratories to experiment with the substance, and various other places to process it, package it, store it, and prepare it for shipment to the market. A typical winery, surrounded by vineyards, may include a mainline brewing facility, a laboratory, a bottling workshop, a storage facility, and a tasting gallery. Fourth, there are stores or outlets to sell the substance; bars, clubs, or restaurants to serve the substance; and employee lounges, shooting galleries, or private corners to take the substance. In some cities, a district, a block, a park, a street, or a facility may be known locally, nationally, or even internationally as a place to buy, exchange, or use a particular substance. Fifth, there are cups, mugs, pipes, matches, lighters, teapots, coffee grinders, glassware, needles, syringes, inhaling devices, and various other substance-specific or nonspecific equipment or tools that are necessary in the process of consumption. Some use equipment is specially made for or is so intertwined with a substance that it eventually becomes an identifier for the substance and its use. An illustrative example is the pipe. It is often taken as an equivalent to tobacco and tobacco use.

Material objects involved in the production, transportation, marketing, and consumption of a substance are essential artifacts in the substance subculture. They not only directly show what a substance is and how it is produced, but also explicitly inform what economic, legal, moral, and social significance a substance has in a particular society or era. A large-scale farming, processing, and manufacturing complex may tell more than statistical numbers about the importance of alcohol or tobacco production in an economy. Late-night bars filled with adults shrouded in smoke and alcoholic smells may say more than words about moral sentiments in a community. Dirty needles and bloody syringes in the corner of a park may convey more than personal stories about the effectiveness or ineffectiveness of the social control or public health authority in a city. Visitors or any novice investigators are likely to learn more from a specialty museum that gathers models, samples, tools, equipment, and other material objects about wine, beer, cigarettes, cigars, coffee, tea, marijuana, cocaine, or heroin, and its respective production and use, than from a monograph that describes and analyzes the same substance with statistics and words.

Nonmaterial Elements

In its nonmaterial aspect, the substance subculture includes knowledge, skills, techniques, beliefs, norms, and rationalizations users develop, share, and accumulate about substance, substance use, substance users, and their collective responses to society. Knowledge divides into general and specific levels. General knowledge concerns various substances with respect to their sources of production, points of supply, forms of consumption, health consequences, legal status, and social reactions. For example, most users, like any average persons in the population, know that marijuana is a controlled substance; it is a plant growing in backyards, farms, or forests; it is purchased in the street; it is smoked; and it is not considered as evil as heroin or cocaine, or that alcohol can be used at certain age; it comes in the form of wine, beer, spirit, and other beverages; it is a depressant; it affects human mobile abilities; and it is available in supermarkets, liquor stores, bars, restaurants, and on many different adult occasions. Specific knowledge regards a particular substance in all its details, from history, name, production, marketing, chemical composition, pharmaceutical properties, routes of administration, metabolic processes, physical and mental symptoms at intake and withdrawal, addiction demographics, treatment methods, and legal definitions, to social control actions. Not every user knows and understands every single detail of the substance he or she takes. But knowledge about various substances and their respective production, consumption, effects on the human body and mind, and impacts over social structure and process grows systematically in the general culture. It essentially shapes the nature of the substance subculture in which individual users find information and support for their habit.

Skills and techniques are useful, sometimes essential, information users need to learn and master in dealing with a substance and its use consequence. While knowledge may be written in the book, skills and techniques may be held only in the hands of individuals. Some have higher skills than others. Some master more sophisticated techniques than others. In securing supply, "A" may be able to obtain a substance at the best possible deal, in terms of originality, purity, quality, potency, and price. In preparing a substance, "B" may be able to identify the most appropriate moment to add or remove something, to heat or cool the mixture, or to take out the final product for serving. In administering a substance, "C" may be able to find the best place to insert the needle, the most proper way to inhale, or the most precise interval to apply a booster dosage so that he or she can maximize the effect of a substance while minimizing substance waste and physical injury. In managing symptoms at intake or withdrawal, "D" may be able to use certain foods, beverages, medicines, body positioning, mind conditioning, environmental backdrops, or exercise to modify, regulate, avoid, or reach a desirable or undesirable mental or physical state. Although many specific skills and techniques are initially explored and developed by individual users, they will eventually become common properties in the substance subculture as users interact with each other and many of them are often eager to validate with other users their individual encounter and experimentation. Even though some of those skills and techniques remain individual idiosyncracies, they logically fall under the substance subculture because users constitute the substance subculture and anything known to users is literally part of it as well.

Beliefs are essential values and points of view held by users about substance and substance-related issues. There are foundation beliefs or philosophical views about the nature of human beings, the equilibrium of the biochemical system, the secrecy of the human mind, the etiology of disease and illness, the power of substance, and the insight of exotic experience. Some may believe that human beings are material beings and substance is an essential agent to bring about change to human experience. Others may argue that ecstacy, fantasy, or transcendency created by substance assists human beings in their search for truth about themselves and the environment in which they live. There are derivative beliefs about or practical approaches to various secular issues on substance. For instance, cigar users believe that cigars are less harmful than cigarettes so that they can smoke more cigars than they would cigarettes. Wine users believe that wine is beneficial so that they can keep wine drinking as a habit. Marijuana growers and users believe that marijuana should not be controlled so that they feel they have a valid reason to hold contempt for those who pursue them in law enforcement and the court. Obviously, beliefs available from the substance subculture about a particular substance and its health, legal, and social aspects can directly or indirectly influence users' attitudes and behavior toward it.

Norms refer to rules and regulations governing users, their behaviors, their interrelations, and their relations with people outside of the substance subculture. There are norms generic to group, organization, and network as the subculture entails bonds, mutual support, and loyalty among its members. Like in any other groupings, members of the substance subculture are supposed to keep secrets from the outside, share information among themselves, protect each other in the face of law enforcement attacks, and condemn, distance, or punish wayward members who break important subcultural norms. For instance, users in the skid row area may gossip about and express their outrage against someone who fails to lend a helping hand to a desperate user, who unjustly takes advantage of a sympathy-worthy user, or who reports critical information about drug dealing in the skid row to the local police. The person may have to leave the area when hostility becomes unbearable. Another major type of norms are those pertinent to substance and substance use. Norms in this category can be based upon knowledge, morality, or both. Knowledge-based norms may dictate: "Never blend substance A with substance B when you serve either substance in a group"; "Have a designated driver when you drink at a party"; and "Call 911 for official assistance when you see that death-signifying symptom in one of your fellow users." Morality-based norms may exclaim: "Always clean used paraphernalia before you hand it over to your fellow user"; "Never offend your buddy by washing a needle/syringe received from him or her"; and "Never call 911 to expose your fellow user if you feel you are able to help him or her with your own hand."

Finally, rationalizations include all excuses, explanations, and justifications users offer about their substance use, usually in response to outside questioning and attack. Rationalizations can be developed on various grounds. In general, there are four major types of rationalizations. Instrumental rationalization focuses on perceived or agreed-upon outcomes substance use brings about to users: "It relieves pain"; "It enhances performance"; and "It relaxes, refreshes, or entertains your mind." Expressive rationalization revolves around emotions, feelings, and sentiments upon which substance use takes place: "I am stressed out"; "I am out of control"; and "It is cool to use it." Traditional rationalization turns to key references for sources of influence in substance use: "I use it as part of a family tradition, back to my parents, my grandparents, and my great grandparents"; "A lot of famous people use it, including movie star A, politician B, and business tycoon C"; and "Almost everyone in my school, my neighborhood, or my company uses it once in a while in his life." The last type is moral rationalization. It appeals to some personal ideals, religious principles, or moral standards users hold about substance, life, or society. For instance, one uses a substance because he or she wants to make a statement about what he or she feels an unjustified control of the substance by the government. One uses a substance in varying dosages because he or she sees his or her use as a sacred mission to explore the diversity of human experience with the substance. And one uses a substance because he or she believes it is a blessing by God or it is a prelude to afterlife.

Relationship to Other Subcultures

The substance subculture follows its individual advocates and practitioners to weave into the whole mosaic of society. In contact with other groups and subcultures, it forges various kinds of external relationships. First, to all other possible subcultures in a society, the substance subculture may find some of them close, similar, friendly, and supportive, some of them remote, different, hostile, and critical, and some of them just irrelevant or nonreactive. Second, the substance subculture cements a cooperative relationship with some other subcultures because it bears with them similar legal or moral attacks from the authority or a same source. For instance, the substance subculture can stand side by side with the crime subculture in resistance against law enforcement, with the prostitute subculture in the face of moral crusade, and with the youth subculture in dealing with social distrust. Third, the substance subculture mingles with some other subcultures when its members cross over different subcultures in their attitudes and behaviors. Youth use psychedelic substances when they curiously explore their body and mind. Seniors count on prescription and over-the-counter drugs when they fearfully crawl through the dusk of their life. Soldiers drink alcohol to boost their courage. AIDS patients smoke marijuana to relieve pain. Homosexuals and prostitutes take methamphetamine to enhance their sexual perfor- mance. Homeless people swallow speed to stay awake. All these mem- ber activities keep the substance subculture inseparable from the youth, elderly, military, AIDS, homosexual, prostitute, and homeless subcultures. Fourth, the substance subculture is drawn into relationship with another subculture because that subculture puts it on notice. For example, although the substance subculture may have no interest in dealing with the subcul- ture of moral crusaders or conservatives, the latter often singles out the former as a menace to or a decay in social morality. As a result, members of the substance subculture may have to come up with some jokes, gestures, or vocabularies to laugh off some of the charges heard from the conserva- tive quarter of society. Finally, the substance subculture is forced into rela- tionship with another subculture when it falls under the jurisdiction or job domain of that subculture. For instance, police officers, drug agents, judges, correctional guards, social workers, counselors, nurses, doctors, and sub- stance abuse researchers approach substance, substance use, and substance users as part of their job duty. They connect the substance subculture to criminal justice, health care, service, and research subcultures as they carry out their work responsibilities on a day-to-day basis.

Relationship to the General Culture

In the sense that various subcultures are part of the general culture, re- lationships the substance subculture establishes with other subcultures al- ready fill in much of the relationship it has with the general culture. Focusing on the information and materials exchanged between the sub- stance culture and other subcultures as well as the general culture, the former not only borrows from, but also contributes to, the latter regard- ing all basic cultural elements, from equipment, materials, artifacts, symbols, language, techniques, and beliefs, to norms. Specifically, the sub- stance culture may buy equipment, such as scales, chemical reaction instruments, and glass containers, from industrial sources, to measure, synthesize, process, transport, and administer a substance. Once a customer-made or modified equipment becomes a fixture in the substance culture, it eventually emerges in the general culture as a new item in the whole inventory of similar equipment. For instance, needle and syringe turn into drug paraphernalia when they are used in drug injection. Drug paraphernalia, as it appears in the general culture, adds drug-blood- tainted syringes and unsafely disposed needles as a new type of use to the repertoire of syringe and needle. Similarly, a bottle becomes a wine bottle in the substance subculture when it is used to hold wine. The wine bottle as a type of bottle represents a unique state of use for bottles in the general culture. The same is true of the teapot, coffee percolator, pipe, and other substance-making or -preparing equipment.

As far as nonmaterial elements are concerned, the substance subculture uses the same language as the general culture. It may invent some special terms, such as joints, pot, ice, and rock, to keep some of its secrets or to symbolize some of its unique features. Some special terms, after long-time use, can gradually become common names for a substance or a type of use in the general culture. For instance, a considerable number of people in the general public know what it means to "smoke pot." The general culture may even tap some of the linguistic inventions from the substance subculture to describe or highlight certain human acts. For instance, people use the power of addiction or obsession transmitted by the term "alcoholic" to coin "workaholic" to refer to someone who works with exceptional devotion and diligence. On the matter of technicality, norm, and morality, knowledge, experience, seniority, faithfulness, loyalty, responsibility, and mutual respect may work in the same spirit in the substance subculture as it does in the general culture. In the context of the substance subculture, each may just take a new form, being more or less intense, genuine, or self-serving. For instance, novice users listen to seasoned users in reaction to law enforcement attacks. Experienced users take care of inexperienced users in the aftermath of a drug overdose. Younger users defer to older users in line for injection or inhalation. Exposed users tell sideline stories or keep their mouth shut to protect their drug use buddies. Ironically and dialectically, the more peculiar some deeds become to the substance subculture, the more likely they arise in the general culture as references to acts of a similar nature. For instance, hallucination is specific to hallucinogens. Codependency is specific to substance-prompted abusive relationships. Tolerance refers to human reactions to a drug and its effects. However, because they each convey powerful images of some unique use states or effects in the substance subculture, they are soon and widely used in the general culture to describe similar acts or situations, such as idealism, illusionism, exploitation, manipulation, fatigue, and trickle-down effect.

Theoretical Applications

In the perspective of subculture, substance, substance use, and substance user can be explored with new light.

A substance may symbolize a subculture. Does it give rise to the subculture or is it a discovery or invention of the subculture? Does it divide or unify members in the subculture? Is it expressively or instrumentally functional to the subculture? Does it glorify or stigmatize the social image of the subculture? A substance may form its own subculture. What explicit material and nonmaterial elements does a substance-specific subculture have? Do material elements of the substance-specific subculture build into established knowledge, production, and service networks? Do nonmaterial elements of the substance-specific subculture mix with dominant social beliefs, norms, and expectations? For instance, the alcohol subculture has grown into many parts of life such that people take alcohol as an essential ingredient in entertainment, party, and social gatherings. A substance may join other substances as part of a large substance subculture. Is it a mild or hard substance? Is it a major or supporting substance? Does it epitomize the large substance subculture or just add some flavor to it?

Substance use, as a culturally embedded act, identifies people. Does it signify people with positive or negative connotation? To what degree does it hide or expose people with regard to their multifaceted identity? With what accuracy does it symbolize people in either the attitudinal or behavioral dimension? For instance, if one uses a substance, how certain and reliable is the prediction that he or she will say certain words or engage in certain activities? Substance use transforms people. Does it bring people together in all main areas of life? To what extent does it affect people in their non-substance-use attitudes or behaviors? Does it entrench people against positive social engagement? For example, if one uses a substance, how likely or probable is the scenario that he or she will turn away from active social life? Substance use reflects social sentiments. Does it signal individual defiance, resistance, or rebellion? Does it convey job stress, normative confusion, cultural intolerance, economic depression, or political repression? Does it point to moral decline, social decay, or general hopelessness? Substance use indicates social needs. Does it call for parental discipline, school prevention, or job counseling? Does it invite law enforcement, medical treatment, or general social intervention? Does it demand deep and sweeping reform in education, social welfare, and justice? For instance, what needs to be done with poverty as substance use is inherently rooted in the culture of poverty? Substance use foretells social change. Does it lead to a culture of abstinence? Does it result in a society of material indulgence? Realistically, how does it influence a society's response to a substance in particular and all substances in general? For example, it is alcohol use in the context of the alcohol subculture that essentially affects people's attitude toward alcohol as well as social definitions of other substances.

Substance users are group actors. Do they physically hang out with each other? Do they reinforce face-to-face contact through telephone, mail, Internet, and other media? Do they focus on use procedure, use rituals, use effect, or some non-substance-use issues in their gatherings? For instance, they meet just to celebrate the release of an album by one of their favorite singers. Substance users are subjects of the substance subculture. What slang, terms, rules, techniques, and artifacts do they create in the main body of the substance subculture? What organizational structure do they put in place in their day-to-day activities? What celebrities or legendary figures do they use as their voices or representatives? What social actions, including public rally, legislative lobbying, and media appearance, do they take to advance their cause? Substance users are objects of the substance subculture. What does each user have to do to gain entry to and become recognized in the substance subculture? How much do individual users matter in the whole dynamics of the substance subculture? What do users need to demonstrate to win social attention, concern, and sympathy? Finally, substance users are collective agents for innovation and rebellion. Are users discoverers of new substances, new uses, and new approaches to material life? Are users explorers of human existence and human potentiality? Are users scouts of life stress and social problems? Are users crusaders against social injustice and repression? For instance, is it possible one day that substance users, acting collectively in the context of the substance subculture, present a new dimension of mind and body functionality otherwise unknown to the general population of material abstinence?

Empirical Tests

The subculture perspective creates opportunities for empirical research on different fronts. Also, it is through various empirical studies that the subculture perspective is tested and confirmed as a credible and useful theoretical framework.

Case studies can target a whole substance subculture or a member of the substance subculture. By examining a substance-specific subculture, such as the tea subculture and the heroin subculture, case studies can gather information on and generate insights about the structure, material and nonmaterial elements, activities, membership, leadership, status system, and evolution of the subculture. In following a user who belongs to a substance subculture, case studies can learn and understand how he or she enters into or exits from the subculture, what he or she gains or loses from the subculture, how he or she relates to other members of the subculture, how he or she proceeds through the system of experience, rank, or status in the subculture, and whether he or she is able to separate his or her engagement in the subculture from his or her other commitments in life.

Historical analysis may focus on the rise and fall of a substance subculture. The subculture may begin with the discovery of a substance and its effects on human beings. It may start off with a group of people who capitalize on the change of law or the shift in morality to advocate for the import and use of a substance. The subculture may sustain well and long due to the substance's natural properties, users' social positions, or its own structural flexibility. It may fall into demise suddenly and instantly because of a replacement substance, a subcultural competitor, or the death of a core of supporters. Historical analysis may ascertain whether an incident triggers a subcultural vogue or a phenomenal subculture tumbles upon a significant event. Historical analysis may also screen out for case studies some users who stay strong above the ups and downs of the subculture pertaining to their substance of choice.

Survey and interview can confront members of the substance subculture with questions on a wide range of issues. Members of the substance subculture may tell their inner experience with the subculture: how much allegiance they hold toward it, what support they obtain from it, what personal freedom they give up for it, what they do with each other, how it affects their world outlook, and how important it is to feel they are part of it. They may provide critical information about specific jargons, symbols, rituals, acts, and codes of conduct: what they mean, how they are spoken or performed, and why they are deemed important to the substance subculture. Survey and interview may also serve as an effective tool to detail users' ambivalence about the general culture. For instance, they may emphasize that they are part of the large culture and that they do not want to be viewed as different, decaying, or rebellious although they remain committed to the substance subculture.

Experimental studies can determine whether the substance subculture is critical to key use decisions: initiation, habituation, or abstinence. Against appropriate control groups, nonusers may be exposed to the substance subculture by watching feature presentations, learning major vocabularies, touring user clubs, attending use ceremonies, visiting treatment programs, or mocking through a typical circle of use. After a designated period of exposure, experimental subjects may be asked about their attitudes toward substance, pointedly: if they decide to stay away from drugs or if they are interested in experimenting with a drug. Regular users may be taken away from their direct use group or environment through experimental research or some natural life events. In a new situation where they have access to their familiar substances but find no support from their familiar substance subculture or face a totally different substance subculture, they may drastically change their use behavior. Finally, pressure from or exposure to a subculture that is squarely opposite to the substance subculture may be examined, through experimental or quasi-experimental designs, to see if it ultimately takes some users to abstinence.

POLICY IMPLICATIONS

The subculture perspective views both substance use and social response to it as culturally embedded behaviors. Such a unique approach has rich implications for substance policies and actions by various social agents and agencies.

Public Health

Public health reactions to substance, substance use, and substance users can lead to different patterns of adaptation from substance users as a cultural collective. Knowledge-based prevention, without moral mandates, may indeed cultivate a sense of self-care, a respect for medical professionals, and an interest in health information among members of the substance subculture. Morality-guided prevention, with limited scientific input, may instead generate suspicion, avoidance, and hostility from substance users toward health workers. Once a general attitudinal and behavioral pattern is established, it tends to reinforce itself toward its own end and completeness. Treatment may result in dependency, loss of self-regulation, recovery, or abstinence. For instance, in-and-out treatment may make substance users feel they can depend upon hospitals and medical professionals as their last resort and ultimate saviors. They take different drugs at one time. They overdose themselves. They experiment with new substances in a knowingly or unknowingly dangerous way. They then count on the medical establishment to clean the mess and bring them back to consciousness. Substance users may also take advantage of some treatment programs to network with one another, to stockpile drug substitutes, to obtain free meals and housing, or just to pass their nonproductive day.

While it is important to understand how substance users collectively respond to public health intervention as a subcultural group, it is equally important to realize how medical response is shaped by the health subculture among medical professionals. There are long-formed and widely spread stereotypes about substance use and substance users. There are newly created and generally known categories for substances and substance use effects. Doctors, nurses, counselors, therapists, and other health workers may joke about substances, symptoms, treatment procedures, and even individual patients with slang, medical jargon, hand signs, facial expressions, or body gestures. They may characterize some drugs as killers, some users as helpless, or some use as suicidal. As most health workers follow their subcultural conventions in dealing with substance use and users, a few may now and then realize that they have to overcome some long-held biases, bypass some taken-for-granted practices, or challenge some seemingly effective measures to achieve truly beneficial prevention or treatment outcomes for their substance use clients.

Social Control

If there are stereotyping and misunderstanding between public health and substance subcultures, there are often clashes and skirmishes between social control and substance use communities. Judges, lawyers, police officers, and other social control agents are each bound by their professional training, organizational conventions, and peer practices. Operating from their respective subculture, they may jump to conclusions about substance use and substance users, without specific inquiry, solid evidence, and serious deliberation. For example, viewing substance users as feeble-minded or untrustworthy, judges may feel inclined to send them to some forcible rehabilitation or supervision programs. Approaching drug addicts as desperate and drug dealers as ruthless, law enforcement agents may stay alert and ready to shoot them during a confrontation or to give them harsh treatment while having them in custody. It is therefore important for social control agents to rise above their own professional subculture and to make case-specific decisions in the spirit of fairness, justice, and humanity.

Social control agents and agencies should also realize that response to their intervention from substance users is often culturally based and supported. In their routine work, social control agents may feel they deal with individual users and case-by-case use incidents. But individual users spread the word within their group and subculture. Particular contacts become contagious through intergroup or intersubculture dynamics. A police officer may soon leave a general impression among users. A justice division or department may soon acquire a public image on the matter of substance and substance use. Once an impression or image is established, it may guide the whole substance use group or subculture in a community in its specific attitudes and behaviors toward social control. Misunderstanding, distrust, hostility, and confrontation can reinforce themselves, turning a community into a battlefield of killing, fear, and horror. Education, persuasion, assistance, and tolerance may also take root, making a district or city a neighborhood of care, support, and cooperation. Between social control and substance use subcultures, the former usually holds the key to a positive, constructive relationship with the latter.

Life and Community

Substance users are not aliens from outer space. They are part of life. They are part of the crowd in the community. What happens in life and in a whole community, materially and nonmaterially, provides fertile soil for sentiments, dispositions, and actions for and against substance use. However, people in the community and the general culture tend to single out deviant groups or subcultures. They often assign labels, shift burdens, or throw blame on those groups for whatever emergencies, crises, or social problems they themselves may actually or ultimately be responsible for. As far as the substance subculture is concerned, although it generally owes the large environment for its own birth and existence, it may instead be condemned and attacked by the general public as an evil source for poverty, moral decay, prostitution, crime, gang warfare, and urban decline. It is thus critically important that people in the community put substance use into perspective and place the substance subculture in historical, legal, moral, political, economic, and social contexts.

Another important insight from the subculture perspective is that life is where substance use comes alive and that community is where substance users connect to their parents, siblings, aunts and uncles, cousins, and friends. Although substance users network with one another in substance use, they interact more extensively and intensively with their family, relative network, and community in many areas of life. Although the substance subculture is attractive to keep substance users in their use habits, the general culture and direct influences from a positive family, kinship, and neighborhood can be more powerful to make people recover from drug dependency and stay free from drugs. The key is that family members, relatives, neighbors, and friends must treat one another with care and respect, influence one another with positive input, and not push one another away in a time of difficulty or on matters of sensitivity. In other words, the substance subculture is given no chance to serve as a surrogate for some individuals to gain their much-needed feelings of sociality, solidarity, belonging, and status.

Work and Organization

The work subculture is general and understandable to most people in society. It features tasks, schedules, rules, deadlines, and achievements. Although it sits well in the mainstream culture, the work subculture can border on and even intersect with the substance subculture in various ways. First, performance demanded at work may prompt substance use. Second, stress generated from the job may lead to substance use. Third, hazards faced at work may require substance-taking treatment or some similar precautionary measures. Fourth, breaks, entertainments, business travels, business occasions, and vacations amid or surrounding work may feature or encourage substance use. When a working individual is interested in a substance or has used a substance, he or she may start making contact with people of the same interest or habit and gathering information about the substance and its use and users. Gradually and naturally, he or she becomes part of the substance subculture. Recognizing the proximity of the work subculture to the substance subculture, people can obviously take proper actions at work if they want to do something about substance use.

An organizational subculture is specific and accessible only to those who are affiliated with it. Depending upon how large it is and where it is located, an organization may dominate a community, with its organizational subculture dictating the general mood of the whole community. It may also just be a tiny unit of a community, with its organizational subculture, if any, being subject to the atmospheric change of the neighborhood. Organizational leaders therefore need to know and understand not only their own organization and organizational culture, but also their large community and community culture. They may find that substance use in the community traces back to some practices or policies in their organization. Or they may find that substance use in their organization is just a spillover of a large social problem in the community. Based upon such a contextual and cultural understanding, they can make more reasonable decisions regarding employees and their fates, or take more effective measures toward substance and substance use in work settings.

In all, the subculture perspective emphasizes substance use as group-based or culturally embedded behavior. Substance can be a symbol used by a group to express its collective views or sentiments. It can also be a cause or source leading to the formation of a whole subculture. Substance use may come from a particular group or be part of a subculture, such as the youth subculture and the prostitute subculture. It may also serve as a base for people from different groups to exchange ideas, to cement relationships, and to improve use practices. Substance users are group actors. They may begin with individual or group initiations. But they all converge in the substance subculture where they affirm use commitment, cultivate motivations, sharpen skills, build networks, develop user identities, and learn how to overcome problems and ward off social attacks.

The substance subculture celebrates and sanctifies substances because it centers on substances. It spreads and sustains substance use because it is shared, learned, and transmitted from individual to individual, group to group, and generation to generation. It protects substance users because it makes them part of a crowd. Individuals make a group but nevertheless cannot be held fully accountable for some group-based actions.

The substance subculture is part of the general culture. It draws spiritual inspiration and material supplies from the general culture. It contributes special symbols, meanings, artifacts, and other residues to the general culture. Although the substance subculture, along with criminal and deviant subcultures, is often singled out for moral condemnation and legal attacks it itself may be a victim of the general failure or crisis in modern and postmodern culture. A holistic approach to substance use and abuse therefore must begin and end with the general social structure and process in the contemporary era.

Conclusion

Having moved through the theoretical jungle of all different sociological perspectives on substance, substance use, and substance users, it is now time to rise above the jungle to see the whole forest and to put the whole intellectual journey into perspective.

First, the book is all based upon existing theories and practices. There is no myth about it. On the theoretical side, all the sociological perspectives included in the book are well-established theories in sociology and criminology. Some of them have even been partially applied to substance use and abuse in specific empirical settings. On the practical side, the book builds upon common knowledge about substance use and general experience from substance users as well as practitioners in substance use counseling and treatment. It does not involve any technical details about particular substances, substance use mechanisms, or substance user groupings.

Second, the book embraces ten different sociological perspectives in its full breadth. It shows that substance, substance use, and substance users can be approached in different ways. One may look at substance use as a complex issue with different facets, such as learning, stress, choice, subculture, and social control aspects. One may look at substance use as a simple subject but nevertheless one that can be examined in different lights, such as career, conflict, functionalist, social disorganization, and social reaction views. Regardless, one can agree that substance use not only looks different, but also plays out differently with different consequences, under different perspectives. Also, juxtaposition of competing perspectives makes people aware that no single view on substance use and abuse is absolute, sacred, ideal, or correct, rightful, and truthful, whether it is imposed by a governing authority, carried on from generation to generation, or fantasized across the populace.

Third, the book delves into each of the ten perspectives in its in-depth exploration. It demonstrates that each perspective is a world of its own. One who abides by a particular perspective can develop his or her own complex of attitudes, patterns of behavior, and mechanisms of adaptation, following the logic of the perspective. Just as presentation of diverse views influences people in their prejudice against substance use and abuse, exposition of one perspective may reinforce people in their adherence to or entrenchment in the perspective, whether they initially lean toward the perspective by way of family, media, or peer influence.

Fourth, the book sets a stage for theorizing and theoretical exploration on substance use and abuse. At the general level, one may ask: why are there only ten different perspectives? Are there any other, more or less insightful, ways to explain and understand substance, substance use, and substance users? Such questions can fuel further explorations for general theories. Specifically, each perspective calls for more substantive work within its conceptual framework. Existing concepts can be refined while new concepts may be identified. Existing theoretical propositions can be fine-tuned while new links may be found and new statements may be made. A real theory can seldom become complete when it is first proposed. It always awaits efforts by numerous enthusiasts to reach its full maturity and potentiality.

Fifth, the book lays ground for empirical research. While each perspective sheds light on existing data, it raises specific questions and creates ample opportunities for testing and substantiation. There are theoretical claims and propositions to be proved or disproved. There are logical links and historical connections to be verified and explored. There are theoretical images and evolutionary patterns to be examined and substantiated. There are predictions and implications to be tested and investigated. All these call for well-reasoned, well-designed, and well-directed research. Compared to practice-prompted studies, theory-induced research possesses greater potential to not only expand and enrich existing methods, but also bring about breakthroughs in general methodology.

Sixth, the book offers intellectual and spiritual inspirations for behavioral modification, practice reform, and policy change. Users may reassess their perceived relationship with a substance, a form of substance use, and a group of fellow users, as well as work, family, community, and general society, and make proper adjustment in their use and nonuse attitudes and behaviors. Practitioners who work with substance users may reflect upon their acquired knowledge through textbooks and their taken-for-granted assumptions, explanations, and treatment regimens from the disciplinary or professional paradigm. A change in approach may not only improve their work, but also raise their clients' hope for a new way of life. Policymakers may pause for a second thought before they act impulsively to condemn and to crusade against substance use and substance users as evil and evildoers. An understanding political atmosphere fosters individual development while promoting social unity. A balanced policy preserves governmental integrity while saving money for taxpayers.

In all, the book serves its purpose if some of its readers, whether they are substance users, people who work with substance users, or people who are generally concerned with substance and its use, say it makes them think again and act differently in their work or habit.

References

Adler, J. 1966. "Gambling, Drugs and Alcohol: A Note on Functional Equivalents." *Issues in Criminology* 2(1): 111–117.

Agnew, R. 1985. "Social Control Theory and Delinquency: A Longitudinal Test." *Criminology* 23: 47–61.

———. 1990. "The Origins of Delinquent Events: An Examination of Offender Accounts." *Journal of Research in Crime and Delinquency* 27(3): 267–294.

Akers, R. L. 1977. *Deviant Behavior: A Social Learning Approach.* Belmont, CA: Wadsworth.

Akers, R. L., and G. Lee. 1996. "A Longitudinal Test of Social Learning Theory: Adolescent Smoking." *Journal of Drug Issues* 26(2): 317–343.

———. 1999. "Age, Social Learning, and Social Bonding in Adolescent Substance Use." *Deviant Behavior* 20(1): 1–25.

Alcoholics Anonymous. 1976. *Alcoholics Anonymous: The Story of How Many Thousands of Men and Women Have Recovered from Alcoholism.* New York: Alcoholics Anonymous World Services.

Andersen, S., and J. E. Berg. 1997. "Rational Drop-Out from Substance Abuse Treatment As a Means to Minimize Personally Felt Risk?" *Addiction Research* 5(6): 507–517.

Anderson, E. 1990. *Streetwise: Race, Class and Change in an Urban Community.* Chicago: University of Chicago Press.

Anderson, N. 1923. *The Hobo: The Sociology of the Homeless Man.* Chicago: University of Chicago Press.

Andrews, J. A., H. Hops, and S. C. Duncan. 1997. "Adolescent Modeling of Parent Substance Use: The Moderating Effect of the Relationship with the Parent." *Journal of Family Psychology* 11(3): 259–270.

Anglin, M. D., M. L. Brecht, and J. A. Woodward. 1986. "An Empirical Study of Maturing Out: Conditional Factors." *International Journal of the Addictions* 21(2): 233–246.

Arrigo, B., and T. Bernard. 1997. "Postmodern Criminology in Relation to Radical and Conflict Criminology." *Critical Criminology* 8: 39–60.

Arthur, M. B., D. T. Hall, and B. S. Lawrence. 1989. *Handbook of Career Theory.* Cambridge: Cambridge University Press.

Auerhahn, K. 1999. "The Split Labor Market and the Origins of Anti-Drug Legislation in the United States." *Law and Social Inquiry* 24(2): 411–440.

Bailey, K. D. 1994. *Methods of Social Research.* New York: Free Press.

Barber, B. 1967. *Drugs and Society.* New York: Russell Sage Foundation.

Barlow, H. 1987. *Introduction to Criminology.* Boston: Little, Brown & Co.

Beccaria, C. 1963. *An Essay on Crimes and Punishments,* translated by H. Paolucci. Indianapolis, IN: Bobbs-Merrill.

Becker, G. S., K. M. Murphy, W. Landes, E. Glaeser, and I. Werning. 2000. *Social Economics: Market Behavior in a Social Environment.* Cambridge, MA: Harvard University Press.

Becker, H. S. 1963. *Outsiders: Studies in the Sociology of Deviance.* New York: Free Press.

Begley, S. 2000. "A World of Their Own." *Newsweek,* May 8: 53–56.

Bell, R., S. Pavis, S. Cunningham-Burley, and A. Amos. 1998. "Young Men's Use of Cannabis: Exploring Changes in Meaning and Context over Time." *Drugs: Education, Prevention and Policy* 5(2): 141–155.

Belsky, J. 1993. "Etiology of Child Maltreatment: A Developmental-Ecological Analysis." *Psychological Bulletin* 114: 413–434.

Benda, B. B. 1999. "Theoretical Model with Reciprocal Effects of Youthful Crime and Drug Use." *Journal of Social Service Research* 25(1–2): 77–107.

Bentham, J. 1843. *Works,* vol. X, edited by J. Bowering. Edinburgh: Tait.

———. 1967. *A Fragment on Government and an Introduction to the Principles of Morals and Legislation,* edited by W. Harrison. Oxford: Basil Blackwell.

Black, D., ed. 1984. *Toward a General Theory of Social Control.* Orlando, FL: Academic Press.

Blumstein, A. 1995. "Youth, Violence, Guns and the Illicit Gun Industry." *Journal of Criminal Law and Criminology* 86: 10–36.

Bonger, W. A. 1916. *Criminality and Economic Conditions,* translated by H. P. Horton. Boston: Little, Brown & Co.

Bordua, D. J. 1959. "Juvenile Delinquency and Anomie: An Attempt at Replication." *Social Problems* 6: 230–238.

Bourgois, P. 1998a. "Families and Children in Pain in the U.S. Inner City." In *Small Wars: The Cultural Politics of Childhood,* edited by N. Scheper-Hughes and C. Sargent. Berkeley: University of California Press.

———. 1998b. "Just Another Night in a Shooting Gallery." *Theory, Culture and Society* 15(2): 37–66.

Brain, K., H. Parker, and T. Carnwath. 2000. "Drinking with Design: Young Drinkers as Psychoactive Consumers." *Drugs: Education, Prevention and Policy* 7(1): 5–20.

Braithwaite, J. 1986. "Retributivism, Punishment, and Privilege." In *Punishment and Privilege,* edited by W. B. Groves and G. Newman. Albany, NY: Harrow & Heston.

———. 1989. *Crime, Shame, and Reintegration.* Melbourne: Cambridge University Press.

Bray, R. M., and M. E. Marsden. 1999. *Drug Use in Metropolitan America*. Thousand Oaks, CA: Sage Publications.

Bronfenbrenner, U. 1977. "Toward an Experimental Ecology of Human Development." *American Psychologist* 32: 513–531.

Burgess, R. L., and R. L. Akers. 1966. "A Differential Association Reinforcement Theory of Criminal Behavior." *Social Problems* 14: 128–147.

Byrne, J., and R. Sampson, eds. 1985. *The Social Ecology of Crime*. New York: Springer Verlag.

Campbell, A. 1984. *The Girls in the Gang*. New York: Basil Blackwell.

Capece, M., and R. L. Akers. 1995. "Supervisor Referrals to Employee Assistance Programs: A Social Learning Perspective." *Journal of Drug Issues* 25(2): 341–361.

Chambliss, W., and R. Seidman. 1971. *Law, Order, and Power*. Reading, MA: Addison-Wesley.

Chamlin, M., and J. Cochran. 1997. "Social Altruism and Crime." *Criminology* 35: 203–227.

Chapin, M. 1994. "Functional Conflict Theory, the Alcohol Beverage Industry, and the Alcoholism Treatment Industry." *Journal of Applied Social Sciences* 18(2): 169–182.

Chen, K., and D. B. Kandel. 1995. "The Natural History of Drug Use from Adolescence to the Mid-Thirties in a General Population Sample." *American Journal of Public Health* 85(1): 41–47.

Chilton, R. J. 1964. "Continuity in Delinquency Area Research: A Comparison of Studies for Baltimore, Detroit and Indianapolis." *American Sociological Review* 29: 11–83.

Cicourel, A. 1968. *The Social Organization of Juvenile Justice*. New York: Wiley.

Clarke, R. 1995. "Situational Crime Prevention." In *Building a Safer Society: Strategic Approaches to Crime Prevention*, edited by M. Tonry and D. Farrington for *Crime and Justice: A Review of Research*, vol. 19. Chicago: University of Chicago Press.

Clarke, R., and R. Homel. 1997. "A Revised Classification of Situational Crime Prevention Techniques." In *Crime Prevention at a Crossroad*, edited by S. Lab. Cincinnati: Anderson.

Clinard, M. B., 1978. *Cities with Little Crime: The Case of Switzerland*. Cambridge: Cambridge University Press.

Clinard, M. B., and D. J. Abbott. 1976. "Community Organization and Property Crime: A Comparative Study of Social Control in the Slums of an African City." In *Delinquency, Crime and Society*, edited by J. F. Short. Chicago: University of Chicago Press.

Cloward, R., and L. Ohlin. 1960. *Delinquency and Opportunity: A Theory of Delinquent Gangs*. New York: Free Press.

Cohen, A. 1955. *Delinquent Boys: The Culture of the Gang*. New York: Free Press.

———. 1965. "The Sociology of the Deviant Act: Anomie Theory and Beyond." *American Sociological Review* 30: 5–14.

Cohen, S., and A. Scull, eds. 1983. *Social Control and the State*. New York: St. Martin's Press.

Combs-Orme, T., J. E. Helzer, and R. H. Miller. 1988. "The Application of Labeling Theory to Alcoholism." *Journal of Social Service Research* 11(2–3): 73–91.

Comte, A. 1896. *The Positive Philosophy*, translated by H. Martineau. London: Bell.

Cook, R. F., A. Back, and J. Trudeau. 1996. "Substance Abuse Prevention in the Workplace: Recent Findings and an Expanded Conceptual Model." *Journal of Primary Prevention* 16(3): 319–339.

Cooley, C. H. 1902. *Human Nature and the Social Order*. New York: Schocken Books, 1964.

Coombs, R. H. 1997. *Drug Impaired Professionals*. Cambridge, MA: Harvard University Press.

Cornish, D., and R. Clarke, eds. 1986. *The Reasoning Criminal: Rational Choice Perspectives on Offending*. New York: Springer Verlag.

Corwyn, R. F., B. B. Benda, and K. Ballard. 1997. "Do the Same Theoretical Factors Explain Alcohol and Other Drug Use among Adolescents?" *Alcoholism Treatment Quarterly* 15(4): 47–62.

Covington, J. 1984. "Insulation from Labeling: Deviant Defenses in Treatment." *Criminology* 22(4): 619–643.

Cressey, P. G. 1932. *The Taxi-Dance Hall: A Sociological Study of Commercialized Recreation and City Life*. Chicago: University of Chicago Press.

Dahrendorf, R. 1959. *Class and Class Conflict in Industrial Society*. Stanford, CA: Stanford University Press.

Daly, K., and M. Chesney-Lind. 1988. "Feminism and Criminology." *Justice Quarterly* 5: 497–538.

Davis, K. 1971. "Prostitution." In *Contemporary Social Problems*, edited by R. K. Merton and R. Nisbet. New York: Harcourt.

Davis, N. J., and B. Anderson. 1983. *Social Control: The Production of Deviance in the Modern State*. New York: Irvington.

Dawes, M., D. Clark, H. Moss, L. Kirisci, and R. Tarter. 1999. "Family and Peer Correlates of Behavioral Self-Regulation in Boys at Risk for Substance Abuse." *American Journal of Drug and Alcohol Abuse* 25(2): 219–237.

Denfield, D., and M. Gordon. 1970. "The Sociology of Mate Swapping: Or the Family that Swings Together Clings Together?" *Journal of Sex Research* 6: 85–100.

Dentler, R. A., and K. T. Erikson. 1959. "The Function of Deviance in Groups." *Social Problems* 7: 98–107.

Donohew, L., R. R. Clayton, W. F. Skinner, and S. Colon. 1999. "Peer Networks and Sensation Seeking: Some Implications for Primary Socialization Theory." *Substance Use and Misuse* 34(7): 1013–1023.

Douglas, J. D. 1977. "Shame and Deceit in Creative Deviance." In *Deviance and Social Change*, edited by E. Sagarin. Beverly Hills, CA: Sage.

Doweiko, H. E. 1996. *Concepts of Chemical Dependency*. Pacific Grove, CA: Brooks/Cole.

Durkheim, E. 1952. *Suicide*, translated by J. A. Spaulding and G. Simpson. New York: Free Press.

———. 1964. *The Rules of the Sociological Method*, translated by S. A. Solovay and J. H. Muller. New York: Macmillan.

Edwards, G., and M. Lader. 1994. *Addiction: Processes of Change*. New York: Oxford University Press.

Elliott, D. S., and H. Voss. 1974. *Delinquent and Dropout*. Lexington, MA: Heath.

Empey, L. T. 1982. *American Delinquency: Its Meaning and Construction*. Homewood, IL: Dorsey.

Ennett, S. T., R. L. Flewelling, R. C. Lindrooth, and E. C. Norton. 1997. "School and Neighborhood Characteristics Associated with School Rates of Alcohol, Cigarette, and Marijuana Use." *Journal of Health and Social Behavior* 38(1): 55–71.

Epstein, J. A., G. J. Botvin, and T. Diaz. 1999. "Social Influence and Psychological Determinants of Smoking among Inner-City Adolescents." *Journal of Child and Adolescent Substance Abuse* 8(3): 1–19.

Erikson, K. T. 1966. *Wayward Puritans: A Study in the Sociology of Deviance*. New York: Wiley.

Esbensen, F. A., and D. S. Elliott. 1994. "Continuity and Discontinuity in Illicit Drug Use: Patterns and Antecedents." *Journal of Drug Issues* 24(1–2): 75–97.

Fagan, J. 1993. "The Political Economy of Drug Dealing among Urban Gangs." Pp. 19–54 in *Drugs and the Community*, edited by R. Davis, A. Lurigio, and D. Rosenbaum. Springfield, IL: Charles C Thomas.

Faris, R. E. L., and H. W. Dunham. 1939. *Mental Disorders in Urban Areas*. Chicago: University of Chicago Press.

Finer, S. E. 1966. *Vilfredo Pareto: Sociological Writings*, translated by D. Mirfin. New York: Praeger.

Franzkowiak, P. 1987. "Risk-Taking and Adolescent Development: The Functions of Smoking and Alcohol Consumption in Adolescence and Its Consequences for Prevention." *Health Promotion* 2(1): 51–61.

Fraser, M., and N. Kohlert. 1988. "Substance Abuse and Public Policy." *Social Service Review* 62(1): 103–126.

Freese, D. E. 1973. "Delinquency, Social Class and the Schools." *Sociology and Social Research* 57: 443–459.

Friedman, S. R., and C. Casriel. 1988. "Drug Users' Organizations and AIDS Policy." *AIDS and Public Policy Journal* 3(2): 30–36.

Furst, R. T., B. D. Johnson, E. Dunlap, and R. Curtis. 1999. "The Stigmatized Image of the 'Crack Head': A Sociocultural Explanation of a Barrier to Cocaine Smoking among a Cohort of Youth in New York City." *Deviant Behavior* 20(2): 153–181.

Garcia, S. A. 1999. "Primary Socialization Theory: Comments on Racism, Sexism, Generational Neglect, Abuse, and Abandonment." *Substance Use and Misuse* 34(7): 1005–1011.

Gardner, E. L. 1992. "Brain Reward Mechanisms." Pp. 70–99 in *Substance Abuse: A Comprehensive Textbook*, edited by J. H. Lowinson, P. Ruiz, and R. B. Millman. Baltimore, MD: Williams & Wilkins.

Gibbs, J. P. 1968. "Crime Punishment and Deterrence." *Social Science Quarterly* 48: 515–530.

———. 1981. *Norms, Deviance, and Social Control*. New York: Elsevier.

Gibbs, J. P., and W. T. Martin. 1964. *Status Integration and Suicide*. Eugene: University of Oregon Press.

Gillin, J. L. 1945. *Criminology and Penology*. New York: Appleton-Century-Crofts.

Glaser, D. 1956. "Criminality Theory and Behavioral Images." *American Journal of Sociology* 61: 433–444.

Glaser, D., B. Lander, and W. Abbott. 1971. "Opiate Addiction and Non-Addicted Siblings in a Slum Area." *Social Problems* 18: 510–521.

Glassner, B., and J. Loughlin. 1987. *Drugs in Adolescent Worlds: Burnouts to Straights*. New York: St. Martin's Press.

Gold, G. 1958. *Theoretical Criminology*. New York: Oxford University Press.

Gold, M. S. 1992. "Cocaine and Crack: Clinical Aspects." Pp. 205–221 in *Substance Abuse: A Comprehensive Textbook*, edited by J. H. Lowinson, P. Ruiz, R. B. Millman, and J. G. Langrod. Baltimore, MD: Williams & Wilkins.

Golub, A., and B. Johnson. 1994. "Cohort Differences in Drug-Use Pathways to Crack among Current Abusers in New York City." *Criminal Justice and Behavior* 21(4): 403–422.

Goode, E. 1994. *Deviant Behavior*. Englewood Cliffs, NJ: Prentice-Hall.

Gordon, D. R. 1994. *The Return of the Dangerous Classes: Drug Prohibition and Policy Politics*. New York: W. W. Norton & Company.

Greenwood, P. 1982. *Selective Incapacitation*. Santa Monica, CA: Rand.

Gropper, M., Z. Liraz, D. Portowicz, and M. Schindler. 1995. "Computer Integrated Drug Prevention: A New Approach to Teach Lower Socioeconomic 5th and 6th Grade Israeli Children to Say No to Drugs." *Social Work in Health Care* 22(2): 87–103.

Hagan, F. E. 2000. *Research Methods in Criminal Justice and Criminology*. Boston: Allyn & Bacon.

Hagan, J. 1989. *Structural Criminology*. New Brunswick, NJ: Rutgers University Press.

Hagedorn, J. M. 1997. "Homeboys, New Jacks, and Anomie." *Journal of African American Men* 3(1): 7–28.

Hall, M. F. 1997. "The 'War on Drugs': A Continuation of the War on the African American Family." *Smith College Studies in Social Work* 67(3): 609–621.

Hanlon, T. E., D. N. Nurco, T. W. Kinlock, and K. R. Duszynski. 1990. "Trends in Criminal Activity and Drug Use over an Addiction Career." *American Journal of Drug and Alcohol Abuse* 16: 223–238.

Harbach, R. L., and W. P. Jones. 1995. "Family Beliefs among Adolescents at Risk for Substance Abuse." *Journal of Drug Education* 25(1): 1–9.

Hassin, J. 1994. "Living a Responsible Life: The Impact of AIDS on the Social Identity of Intravenous Drug Users." *Social Science and Medicine* 39(3): 391–400.

Hathaway, A. D. 1997. "Marijuana and Tolerance: Revisiting Becker's Sources of Control." *Deviant Behavior* 18(2): 103–124.

Hayner, N. 1936. *Hotel Life*. Chicago: University of Chicago Press.

Henry, A., and J. F. Short. 1954. *Suicide and Homicide*. Glencoe, IL: Free Press.

Higgins, P. C., G. L. Albrecht, and M. H. Albrecht. 1977. "Black-White Adolescent Drinking: The Myth and the Reality." *Social Problems* 25(2): 215–224.

Hirschi, T. 1969. *Causes of Delinquency*. Los Angeles: University of California Press.

Hoffmann, J. P. 2000. "Introduction to the Special Issue on Stress and Substance Use." *Substance Use and Misuse* 35(5): 635–641.

Hoffmann, J. P., and S. S. Su. 1997. "The Conditional Effects of Stress on Delinquency and Drug Use: A Strain Theory Assessment of Sex Differences." *Journal of Research in Crime and Delinquency* 34: 46–78.

Holloway, L. 1998. "Teacher Threatened over Book Weighs Switching Schools." *New York Times*, November 27: 1A.

Horton, D. 1943. "Functions of Alcohol in Primitive Societies." *Quarterly Journal of Studies in Alcohol* 4: 199–320.

Horwitz, A. 1990. *The Logic of Social Control*. New York: Plenum.

Inciardi, J. A. 1992. *The War on Drugs II: The Continuing Epic of Heroin, Cocaine, Crack, Crime, AIDS, and Public Policy*. Mountain View, CA: Mayfield.

Jaffe, J. H. 1992. "Opiates: Clinical Aspects." In *Substance Abuse: A Comprehensive Textbook*, edited by J. H. Lowinson, P. Ruiz, R. B. Millman, and J. G. Langrod. Baltimore, MD: Williams & Wilkins.

Janes, C. R., and G. Ames. 1989. "Men, Blue Collar Work and Drinking: Alcohol Use in an Industrial Subculture." *Culture, Medicine and Psychiatry* 13(3): 245–274.

Janowitz, M. 1975. "Sociological Theory and Social Control." *American Journal of Sociology* 81(1): 82–108.

Jensen, G. F., J. H. Stauss, and W. V. Harris. 1977. "Crime, Delinquency, and the American Indian." *Human Organization* 36(3): 252–257.

Johnson, B. R., D. B. Larson, S. D. Li, and S. J. Jang. 2000. "Escaping from the Crime of Inner Cities: Church Attendance and Religious Salience among Disadvantaged Youth." *Justice Quarterly* 17(2): 377–391.

Jones, C. L., and C. S. Bell-Bolek. 1986. "Kids and Drugs: Why, When, and What Can We Do about It?" *Children Today* 15: 5–10.

Kandel, D. B., K. Yamaguchi, and K. Chen. 1992. "Stages of Progression in Drug Involvement from Adolescence to Adulthood: Further Evidence for the Gateway Theory." *Journal of Studies on Alcohol* 53: 447–457.

Kaplan, H. B. 1987. "Social Sanctions, Self-Referent Responses, and the Continuation of Substance Abuse: A Person-Environment Interaction Perspective." *Drugs and Society* 2(1): 31–55.

Kaplan, H. B., and H. Fukurai. 1992. "Negative Social Sanctions, Self-Rejection, and Drug Use." *Youth and Society* 23(3): 275–298.

Kerr, J. S. 1996. "Two Myths of Addiction: The Addictive Personality and the Issue of Free Choice." *Human Psychopharmacology—Clinical and Experimental* 11(1): 9–13.

Khalsa, M. E., A. Paredes, and M. D. Anglin. 1993. "Cocaine Dependence: Behavioral Dimensions and Patterns of Progression." *American Journal on Addictions* 2(4): 330–345.

Kleiman, M. 1992–1993. "Drug Abuse Control Policy: Libertarian, Authoritarian, Liberal, and Communitarian Perspectives." *The Responsive Community* 3(1): 44–53.

Knight, D. K., K. M. Broome, D. R. Cross, and D. D. Simpson. 1998. "Antisocial Tendency among Drug-Addicted Adults: Potential Long-Term Effects of Parental Absence, Support, and Conflict during Childhood." *American Journal of Drug and Alcohol Abuse* 24(3): 361–375.

Knipe, E. 1995. *Culture, Society, and Drugs: The Social Science Approach to Drug Use*. Prospect Heights, IL: Waveland Press.

Korem, D. 1994. *Suburban Gangs: Affluent Rebels*. Richardson, TX: International Focus.

Kornhauser, R. 1978. *Social Sources of Delinquency*. Chicago: University of Chicago Press.

Krohn, M. D., and J. L. Massey. 1980. "Social Control and Delinquent Behavior: An Examination of the Elements of the Social Bond." *Sociological Quarterly* 21: 529–544.

Lander, B. 1954. *Towards an Understanding of Juvenile Delinquency*. New York: Columbia University Press.

Lea, J., and J. Young. 1984. *What Is To Be Done about Law and Order?* Harmondsworth, UK: Penguin.

League of Nations. 1930. *Opium and Other Dangerous Drugs*. Geneva: Commission of Enquiry into the Control of Opium-Smoking in the Far East.

Lemert, E. 1951. *Social Pathology*. New York: McGraw-Hill.

Lewis, D. C., D. F. Duncan, and P. R. Clifford. 1997. "Analyzing Drug Policy." *Journal of Primary Prevention* 17(4): 351–361.

Lewis, M. 1970. "Structural Deviance and Normative Conformity: The 'Hustle' and the 'Gang.'" In *Crime in the City*, edited by D. Glaser. New York: Harper & Row.

Lindesmith, A. R., and J. H. Simon. 1964. "Anomie and Drug Addiction." Pp. 158–188 in *Anomie and Deviant Behavior*, edited by M. B. Clinard. New York: Free Press.

Lindstrom, L. 1987. *Drugs in Western Pacific Societies: Relations of Substance*. Lanham, MD: University Press of America.

Lowinson, J. H., P. Ruiz, R. B. Millman, and J. G. Langrod, eds. 1992. *Substance Abuse: A Comprehensive Textbook*. Baltimore, MD: Williams & Wilkins.

Makela, K., and H. Mustonen. 2000. "Relationships of Drinking Behaviour, Gender and Age with Reported Negative and Positive Experiences Related to Drinking." *Addiction* 95(5): 727–736.

Maris, R. W. 1969. *Social Forces in Urban Suicide*. Homewood, IL: Dorsey.

Marlatt, G. A., and G. R. VandenBos, eds. 1997. *Addictive Behavior: Readings on Etiology, Prevention, and Treatment*. Washington, DC: American Psychological Association.

Marx, K., and F. Engels. 1979. *The Communist Manifesto*. New York: International Publishers, 1848.

Matza, D. 1964. *Delinquency and Drift*. New York: Wiley.

Maurer, D. W., and V. H. Vogel. 1954. *Narcotics and Narcotic Addiction*. Springfield, IL: Charles C Thomas.

Mazerolle, L. G., C. Kadleck, and J. Roehl. 1998. "Controlling Drug and Disorder Problems: The Role of Place Managers." *Criminology* 36(2): 371–404.

McGee, Z. T. 1992. "Social Class Differences in Parental and Peer Influence on Adolescent Drug Use." *Deviant Behavior* 13: 349–372.

Meier, K. J. 1994. *The Politics of Sin: Drugs, Alcohol, and Public Policy*. Armonk, NY: M. E. Sharpe.

Meints, J. 1979. "Labeling, the Career Methadone Patient, and the Clinical Rehabilitation Process." *California Sociologist* 2(2): 165–180.

Merton, R. K. 1938. "Social Structure and Anomie." *American Sociological Review* 3: 672–682.

———. 1957. *Social Theory and Social Structure*. New York: Free Press.

_____. 1968. *Social Theory and Social Structure*. Enlarged edition. New York: Free Press.

Michalowski, R. 1977. "The Social and Criminal Patterns of Urban Traffic Fatalities." *British Journal of Criminology* 17(2): 126–140.

Mider, P. A. 1983. "Personality Typologies of Addicts by Drug of Choice." *Bulletin of the Society of Psychologists in Addictive Behaviors* 2(3): 197–217.

Miller, R. L. 1996. *Drug Warriors and Their Prey: From Police Power to Police State*. Westport, CT: Praeger.

Miller, W. 1958. "Lower Class Culture as a Generating Milieu of Gang Delinquency." *Journal of Social Issues* 14: 5–19.

Morales, E. 1986. "Coca Paste and Crack: A Cross National Ethnographic Approach." *Studies in Third World Societies* 37: 179–200.

Mowner, E. 1927. *Family Disorganization*. Chicago: University of Chicago Press.

Musto, D. F. 1999. *The American Disease: Origins of Narcotic Control*. New York: Oxford University Press.

Niesink, R. J. M., R. M. A. Jaspers, L. M. W. Kornet, and J. M. van Ree. 1999. *Drugs of Abuse and Addiction: Neurobehavioral Toxicology*. Boca Raton, FL: CRC Press.

Noguera, P., and P. Morgan. 1993–1994. "Taking Chances, Taking Charge: A Report on a Drug Abuse Intervention Conceived, Created and Controlled by a Community." *International Quarterly of Community Health Education* 14(4): 417–433.

Park, R. E. 1936. "Human Ecology." *American Journal of Sociology* 42: 1–15.

Park, R. E., E. W. Burgess, and R. D. McKenzie. 1967. *The City*. Chicago: University of Chicago Press.

Parsons, T. 1951. *The Social System*. New York: Free Press.

Pepinsky, H., and R. Quinney. 1991. *Criminology as Peacemaking*. Bloomington: Indiana University Press.

Piliavin, I., and S. Briar. 1964. "Police Encounters with Juveniles." *American Journal of Sociology* 70: 206–214.

Powis, B., M. Gossop, C. Bury, K. Payne, and P. Griffiths. 2000. "Drug-Using Mothers: Social, Psychological and Substance Use Problems of Women Opiate Users with Children." *Drug and Alcohol Review* 19(2): 171–180.

Quinney, R. 1975. "Crime Control in Capitalist Society." In *Critical Criminology*, edited by I. Taylor, P. Walton, and J. Young. London: Routledge & Kegan Paul.

Ray, M. C., and W. R. Downs. 1986. "An Empirical Test of Labeling Theory Using Longitudinal Data." *Journal of Research in Crime and Delinquency* 23(2): 169–194.

Ray, O., and C. Ksir. 1996. *Drugs, Society, and Human Behavior*. St. Louis, MO: Mosby.

Reckless, W. C. 1961. "A New Theory of Delinquency and Crime." *Federal Probation* 25: 42–46.

_____. 1962. "A Non-Causal Explanation: Containment Theory." *Excerpta Criminologia* 2: 131–132.

Reiss, A. J. 1951. "Delinquency as the Failure of Personal and Social Controls." *American Sociological Review* 16: 206.

Renard, R. D. 1996. *The Burmese Connection: Illegal Drugs and the Making of the Golden Triangle*. Boulder, CO: L. Rienner Publishers.

Ridlon, F. 1988. *A Fallen Angel: The Status Insularity of the Female Alcoholic*. Lewisburg, PA: Bucknell University Press.

Ringwalt, C. L., J. M. Greene, and M. J. Robertson. 1998. "Familial Backgrounds and Risk Behaviors of Youth with Thrownaway Experiences." *Journal of Adolescence* 21(3): 241–252.

Ronel, N. 1998. "Narcotics Anonymous: Understanding the 'Bridge of Recovery.'" *Journal of Offender Rehabilitation* 27(1–2): 179–197.

Ross, E. A. 1901. *Social Control: A Survey of the Foundations of Order*. New York: Macmillan.

Roucek, J. S., ed. 1978. *Social Control for the 1980s: A Handbook for Order in a Democratic Society*. Westport, CT: Greenwood Press.

Rowe, D. C., and B. L. Gulley. 1992. "Sibling Effects on Substance Use and Delinquency." *Criminology* 30(2): 217–233.

Rusche, G., and O. Kirchheimer. 1939. *Punishment and Social Structure*. New York: Columbia University Press.

Scheier, L. M., and G. J. Botvin. 1996. "Purpose in Life, Cognitive Efficacy, and General Deviance as Determinants of Drug Abuse in Urban Black Youth." *Journal of Child and Adolescent Substance Abuse* 5(1): 1–26.

Scheier, L. M., G. J. Botvin, and N. L. Miller. 1999. "Life Events, Neighborhood Stress, Psychological Functioning, and Alcohol Use among Urban Minority Youth." *Journal of Child and Adolescent Substance Abuse* 9(1): 19–50.

Schultes, R. E., and A. Hofmann. 1979. *Plants of the Gods*. New York: McGraw-Hill.

Schur, E. 1973. *Radical Non-Intervention: Rethinking the Delinquency Problem*. Englewood Cliffs, NJ: Prentice-Hall.

Schwartz, M., and W. DeKeseredy. 1993. *Contemporary Criminology*. Belmont, CA: Wadsworth.

Schwendinger, H., and J. S. Schwendinger. 1985. *Adolescent Subcultures and Delinquency*. New York: Praeger.

Sebald, H. 1968. *Adolescence: A Sociological Analysis*. New York: Appleton-Century-Crofts.

Sellers, C. S., and L. T. Winfree. 1990. "Differential Associations and Definitions: A Panel Study of Youthful Drinking Behavior." *International Journal of the Addictions* 25(7): 755–771.

Sellin, T. 1938. "Culture, Conflict and Crime." *Bulletin* 41. Washington, DC: Social Science Research Council.

Sharp, S. F., T. L. Terling-Watt, L. A. Atkins, J. T. Gilliam, and A. Sanders. 2001. "Purging Behavior in a Sample of College Females: A Research Note on General Strain and Female Deviance." *Deviant Behavior* 22(2): 171–188.

Shaw, C. R. 1930. *The Jack Roller: A Delinquent Boy's Own Story*. Chicago: University of Chicago Press.

Shaw, C. R., F. M. Forgaugh, H. D. McKay, and L. S. Cottreel. 1929. *Delinquency Areas*. Chicago: University of Chicago Press.

Shaw, C. R., and J. F. McDonald. 1938. *Brothers in Crime*. Chicago: University of Chicago Press.

Shaw, C. R., and H. D. McKay. 1969. *Juvenile Delinquency and Urban Areas: A Study of Rates of Delinquency in Relation to Differential Characteristics of Local Communities in American Cities.* Chicago: University of Chicago Press.

Shaw, C. R., and M. Moore. 1931. *The Natural History of a Delinquent Career.* Chicago: University of Chicago Press.

Shaw, V. N. 1996. *Social Control in China: A Study of Chinese Work Units.* Westport, CT: Greenwood Publishing Group.

———. 1999. "Toward a Systematic Understanding: A Two-Way Relational Model between Drug Use and HIV/AIDS." *AIDS and Public Policy Journal* 14(1): 30–43.

Shaw, V. N., Y. I. Hser, M. D. Anglin, and K. Boyle. 1999. "Sequences of Powder Cocaine and Crack Use among Arrestees in Los Angeles County." *American Journal of Drug and Alcohol Abuse* 25(1): 47–66.

Sheleff, L. S. 1981. "The Relevance of Classical Criminology Today." In *The Mad, the Bad, and the Different: Essays in Honor of Simon Dinitz,* edited by I. L. Barak-Glantz and C. R. Huff. Lexington, MA: Lexington Books.

Shoemaker, D. J. 1984. *Theories of Delinquency: An Examination of Explanations of Delinquent Behavior.* New York: Oxford University Press.

Skinner, B. F. 1953. *Science and Human Behavior.* New York: Macmillan.

Smith, E. A. 1962. *American Youth Culture.* Glencoe, IL: Free Press.

Snyder, C. 1964. "Inebriety, Alcoholism, and Anomie." In *Anomie and Deviant Behavior,* edited by M. Clinard. Glencoe, NY: Free Press.

Sollenberger, R. T. 1968. "Chinese-American Child-Rearing Practices and Juvenile Delinquency." *Journal of Social Psychology* 74(1): 13–23.

Spencer, H. 1896. *The Principle of Sociology.* New York: Appleton.

Spitzer, S. 1975. "Toward a Marxian Theory of Deviance." *Social Problems* 22: 641–651.

Spotts, J. V., and F. C. Shontz. 1985. "A Theory of Adolescent Substance Abuse." *Advances in Alcohol and Substance Abuse* 4(3–4): 117–138.

Strang, J., and G. V. Stimson, eds. 1990. *AIDS and Drug Misuse: The Challenge for Policy and Practice in the 1990s.* London: Routledge.

Sussman, S., and C. W. Dent. 2000. "One-Year Prospective Prediction of Drug Use from Stress-Related Variables." *Substance Use and Misuse* 35(5): 717–735.

Sutherland, E. H. 1934. *Principles of Criminology.* Philadelphia: Lippincott.

———. 1937. *The Professional Thief.* Chicago: University of Chicago Press.

———. 1947. *Principles of Criminology.* 4th ed. Philadelphia: Lippincott.

Sutter, A. 1972. "Play a Cold Game: Phases of a Ghetto Career." *Urban Life and Culture* 1(1): 77–91.

Svensson, R. 2000. "Risk Factors for Different Dimensions of Adolescent Drug Use." *Journal of Child and Adolescent Substance Abuse* 9(3): 67–90.

Sykes, G., and D. Matza. 1957. "Techniques of Neutralization: A Theory of Delinquency." *American Sociological Review* 22: 664–670.

Tannenbaum, F. 1938. *Crime and the Community.* Boston: Ginn & Co.

Tarde, G. 1912. *Penal Philosophy.* Boston: Little, Brown & Co.

Tarter, R. E., and M. Vanyukov. 1994. "Alcoholism: A Developmental Disorder." *Journal of Consulting and Clinical Psychology* 62: 1096–1107.

Taylor, I., P. Walton, and J. Young. 1973. *The New Criminology: For a Social Theory of Deviance.* London: Routledge and Kegan Paul.

Taylor, R., and J. Covington. 1988. "Neighborhood Changes in Ecology and Violence." *Criminology* 26: 553–589.

———. 1993. "Community Structural Change and Fear of Crime." *Social Problems* 40: 374–392.

Thomas, E. 1986. "America's Crusade: What Is behind the Latest War on Drugs?" *Time* 128: 60–68.

Thomas, W. I. 1923. *The Unadjusted Girl*. Boston: Little, Brown & Co.

———. 1931. *The Unadjusted Girl*. Revised ed. Boston: Little, Brown & Co.

Thomas, W. I., and F. Znaniecki. 1920. *The Polish Peasant in Europe and America*. Boston: Gorham Press.

Thrasher, F. M. 1927. *The Gang*. Chicago: University of Chicago Press.

Tifft, L., and D. Sullivan. 1980. *The Struggle To Be Human: Crime, Criminology, and Anarchism*. Orkney, Scotland: Cienfuegos Press.

Toby, J. 1957. "Social Disorganization and Stake in Conformity: Complementary Factors in the Predatory Behavior of Hoodlums." *Journal of Criminal Law, Criminology, and Police Science* 48: 12–17.

Triplett, R., and G. R. Jarjoura. 1997. "Specifying the Gender-Class Relationship: Exploring the Effects of Educational Expectations." *Sociological Perspectives* 40(2): 287–316.

Turk, A. 1969. *Criminality and Legal Order*. Chicago: Rand McNally.

U.S. Department of Health and Human Services. 1993. *National Household Survey on Drug Abuse*. Rockville, MD: DHHS Publication 93–2053.

Usher, M. L. 1991. "From Identification to Consolidation: A Treatment Model for Couples and Families Complicated by Alcoholism." *Family Dynamics of Addiction Quarterly* 1(2): 45–58.

Venkatesh, S. A. 1996. "The Gang in the Community." In *Gangs in America*, edited by C. R. Huff. Thousand Oaks, CA: Sage Publications.

Volkman, R., and D. R. Cressey. 1963. "Differential Association and the Rehabilitation of Drug Addicts." *American Journal of Sociology* 69: 129–142.

Waldorf, D. 1983. "Natural Recovery from Opiate Addiction: Some Social-Psychological Processes of Untreated Recovery." *Journal of Drug Issues* 2: 237–280.

Wallace, R. A., and A. Wolf. 1995. *Contemporary Sociological Theory: Continuing the Classical Tradition*. Englewood Cliffs, NJ: Prentice-Hall.

Wallerstedt, J. 1984. *Returning to Prison*. Washington, DC: U.S. Department of Justice.

Walshak, M. L. 1971. "The Emergence of Middle-Class Deviant Subcultures: The Case of Swingers." *Social Problems* 18: 488–495.

Walters, G. D. 1994. *Drugs and Crime in Lifestyle Perspective*. Thousand Oaks, CA: Sage Publications.

Walton, J. A. 1992. "Attitudes among College Students as They Apply to Labeling the Alcoholic/Problem Drinker." *Free Inquiry in Creative Sociology* 20(2): 217–222.

Ward, D. A., and C. R. Tittle. 1993. "Deterrence or Labeling: The Effects of Informal Sanctions." *Deviant Behavior: An Interdisciplinary Journal* 14: 43–64.

Weinberg, S. K. 1976. "Shaw-McKay Theories of Delinquency in Cross Cultural Context." Pp. 167–185 in *Delinquency, Crime and Society*, edited by J. F. Short. Chicago: University of Chicago Press.

Whyte, W. F. 1943. *Street Corner Society: The Social Structure of an Italian Slum.* Chicago: University of Chicago Press.

Williams, J. R. 1976. *Effects of Labeling the "Drug-Abuser": An Inquiry.* Rockville, MD: National Institute on Drug Abuse.

Wilson, J. Q. 1975. *Thinking about Crime.* New York: Vintage.

Wilson, W. J. 1987. *The Truly Disadvantaged.* Chicago: University of Chicago Press.

Winfree, L. T., C. S. Sellers, and D. L. Clason. 1993. "Social Learning and Adolescent Deviance Abstention: Toward Understanding the Reasons for Initiating, Quitting, and Avoiding Drugs." *Journal of Quantitative Criminology* 9(1): 101–125.

Wirth, L. 1928. *Ghetto.* Chicago: University of Chicago Press.

———. 1931. "Culture Conflict and Misconduct." *Social Forces* 9(4): 484–492.

Wolfgang, M. E., and F. Ferracuti. 1967. *The Subculture of Violence: Toward an Integrated Theory in Criminology.* London: Tavistock.

Wolfgang, M. E., R. Figlio, and T. Sellin. 1972. *Delinquency in a Cohort.* Chicago: University of Chicago Press.

Zack, M., and M. Vogel-Sprott. 1997. "Drunk or Sober? Learned Conformity to a Behavioral Standard." *Journal of Studies on Alcohol* 58(5): 495–501.

Zimny, M. J. 2000. "Alcoholism and Morality in Poland and Eastern Europe: The Social Consequences of Democratization." *Dissertation Abstracts International* 61(5): 2060–2061.

Zorbaugh, H. W. 1929. *Gold Coast and Slum.* Chicago: University of Chicago Press.

Index

About the Author

VICTOR N. SHAW is Assistant Professor, Department of Sociology, California State University, Northridge.

DISCARD